SpringerWienNewYork

Stephan Becker
Michael Ogon (Eds.)

Balloon Kyphoplasty

SpringerWienNewYork

Dr. med. Stephan Becker
Univ.-Doz. Dr. med. Michael Ogon
Wirbelsäulenzentrum, 3. Orthopädische Abteilung, Orthopädisches Spital Speising, Vienna, Austria

This work is subject to copyright.
All rights are reserved, whether the whole or part of the material is concerned, specifically those of translation, reprinting, re-use of illustrations, broadcasting, reproduction by photocopying machines or similar means, and storage in data banks. Product Liability: The publisher can give no guarantee for all the information contained in this book. This does also refer to information about drug dosage and application thereof. In every individual case the respective user must check its accuracy by consulting other pharmaceutical literature. The use of registered names, trademarks, etc. in this publication does not imply, even in the absence of a specific statement, that such names are exempt from the relevant protective laws and regulations and therefore free for general use.

© 2008 Springer-Verlag/Wien
Printed in Austria
SpringerWienNewYork is a part of
Springer Science + Business Media
springer.at

Typesetting: Grafik Rödl, 2486 Pottendorf, Austria
Printing: Druckerei Theiss GmbH, 9431 St. Stefan, Austria

Printed on acid-free and chlorine-free bleached paper
SPIN: 11906520

With 121 (partly coloured) Figures

Library of Congress Control Number: 2007940957

ISBN   978-3-211-74220-4   SpringerWienNewYork

Preface

Osteoporosis is one of the ten most important diseases worldwide and its importance will rise further following the aging of the population. Vertebral fractures are the most common fractures in osteoporosis and have significant impact on quality of life and survival rates, as well as carrying increased socioeconomic costs.

The establishment of minimally invasive treatment schemes in recent years has led to reduced perioperative morbidity and increased early mobilization. This book focuses on balloon kyphoplasty and alternative minimally invasive treatments for stabilization of osteoporotic vertebral fractures.

The optimal treatment of a patient with osteoporotic vertebral fractures requires an interdisciplinary approach, and therefore our book draws on the expertise of orthopedic surgeons, traumatologists and neurosurgeons, and also includes a chapter on medical treatment.

We are happy to present the first English edition of this book. All chapters have been extensively revised and updated. In addition to a detailed description of the technique of balloon kyphoplasty, with practical tips from experts, the book retains a chapter on the medical treatment of osteoporosis, which is still indispensable in the interdisciplinary approach to osteoporosis. This well established concept, uniting several treatment aspects including conservative treatment, is preserved in this book. However, new chapters have been added as the result of recent developments and clinical findings. These include a new step-by-step treatment scheme for osteoporosis, new clinical and biomechanical aspects, and a chapter on special indications such as osteonecrosis. Furthermore an entire new chapter discussing the indication and clinical results of balloon kyphoplasty in trauma has been added.

In keeping with the international aspect of this book, the reimbursement schemes of several countries have been added in order to provide insight into current reimbursement strategies.

Stephan Becker and *Michael Ogon*

Contents

Contributors IX

Acknowledgement XI

Chapter 1. Epidemiology of osteoporosis (S. Becker and M. Ogon) 1
Incidence and prevalence of vertebral fractures 1
Sex differences 2
Socio-economic consequences 2

Chapter 2. Drug therapy of osteoporosis (H. Resch and C. Muschitz) 5
Pathogenic mechanism and pharmacological effects 5
Therapeutic goals 6
    1) The treatment of pain 6
    2) Reduction of the risk of fracture 6
    3) Increase of bone density 6
    4) Influencing biochemical markers of bone metabolism 6
Indication for osteoporosis therapy 7
Treatment options 7
    Basic medication with calcium-vitamin D 7
        Calcium 7
    The combination of calcium with vitamin D 8
    Hormone replacement therapy – a fundamental change in evaluation 8
    Substances that inhibit bone absorption 9
        Bisphosphonates 9
    Selective estrogen-receptor modulators 10
    Calcitonins 10
    Tibolone 10
    Substances that increase bone formation 10
        Parathormone 10
    Combination therapies 10
    Parathormone and antiresorptives 11
    Fluorides 11
    Substances with a synchronous effect on bone formation and absorption 11
    Substances with a biological effect 11
        The RANKL antibody – new approaches in the treatment of osteoporosis 11
Osteoporosis in men 12
    Prevention and therapy 12

Chapter 3. Clinical aspects and mortality risk of the osteoporotic spine fracture (S. Becker and M. Ogon) 17
Clinical diagnosis of spinal fracture 17
The clinical consequences of a spinal fracture 18
Mortality after fractures of the spine 19

Chapter 4. Biomechanics 23
Biomechanics of cement injection in vertebroplasty (G. Baroud and A. Schleyer) 23
    Summary 23
    Introduction 23
    In vivo measurements of injection pressure/volume versus time for three representative cases of vertebroplasty .. 24
    Analysis of injection pressures during vertebroplasty 25
    Experimental determination of the different pressure components during a cement injection 26
    Analysis of risk of cement extravasation out of the vertebral body 27

VIII   Contents

Development of a new injection cannula   28
Conclusions   29
Acknowledgments   30
Glossary   30
Biomechanics of vertebral cement augmentation: risk of adjacent fractures following vertebroplasty
(G. Baroud and S. Wolf)   31
Summary   31
Introduction   31
Methods and results   31
Discussion   36

Chapter 5. Indications, contraindications and imaging in balloon kyphoplasty (S. Becker)   39

Indications and contraindications   39
Imaging   39
Sequential therapy after osteoporotic vertebral fracture – a treatment scheme   41

Chapter 6. Special anatomy and classification of fractures   45

The venous drainage system of the vertebral body and spine and its consequences for balloon kyphoplasty
(S. Becker)   45
The vertebral venous system   45
The basivertebral system   45
The internal vertebral venous system   46
Classification of osteoporotic vertebral fractures (B. Boszczyk)   47

Chapter 7. The technique of balloon kyphoplasty (S. Becker)   49

The set of instruments   49
The balloon catheter (inflatable) bone tamp and the pressure syringe   50
Anatomical landmarks and image intensifier settings   51
The pedicles   51
The spinous process   51
The endplates and the posterior wall   51
Special procedures in the case of scoliosis   52
Starting and end points in lumbar transpedicular operations   52
Starting point   52
End points   53
Starting and end points in thoracic extrapedicular operations   55
Preparation and positioning of the patient   56
Performing balloon kyphoplasty   56
The impact of positioning versus balloon kyphoplasty on restoration of vertebral height   56
Anesthesiological preparation   56
Lumbar transpedicular access   57
Extrapedicular access   64
Malpositioning of the working cannula   65
High thoracic approach (B. Boszczyk)   66
Instructions for preparation of the cement (S. Becker)   69
Radiation exposure (B. Boszczyk and M. Bierschneider)   70

Chapter 8. Results in kyphoplasty, risks and complications (U. Berlemann, P. Hulme, and O. Schwarzenbach) . . .   73

Materials and methods   73
Results   74
Pain relief   74
Correction of kyphosis   74
Complications   74
New fractures   74
Discussion   76
Summary: the risks of kyphoplasty (M. Bierschneider, B. Boszczyk, and H. Jaksche)   79
1. Preoperative risks   79

Contents IX

2. Intraoperative risks 79
3. Postoperative risks 83
Conclusion 83

Chapter 9. Special indications and techniques of balloon kyphoplasty (S. Becker and M. Ogon) 85

Balloon kyphoplasty for the treatment of malignant bone tumors 85
    Plasmocytoma (multiple myeloma) 85
    Osteolytic metastases 85
    Special techniques in cases of plasmocytoma (multiple myeloma) and osteolytic metastases 88
Microsurgical interlaminary balloon kyphoplasty (B. Boszczyk and M. Bierschneider) 90
Special balloon kyphoplasty techniques in cases of screw loosening and in spinal defects (S. Becker and M. Ogon) . . . 93
    Transpedicular balloon kyphoplasty after screw removal 93
    Augmentation techniques 93
    The egg-shell technique 93
    Support technique 93
The treatment of vertebral osteonecrosis and vertebra plana with balloon kyphoplasty (S. Becker) 98

Chapter 10. Indications and experience with balloon kyphoplasty in trauma 105

Balloon-assisted endplate reduction combined with vertebroplasty for the treatment of traumatic vertebral body
fractures (J.-J. Verlaan, W. J. A. Dhert, and F. Cumhur Oner) 105
    Current approaches and techniques for the treatment of traumatic vertebral fractures 105
    Experimental and clinical studies for the development of transpedicular augmentation techniques of the anterior
    spinal column in traumatic fractures 106
        First steps in developing a direct reduction technique for burst fractures 106
        The choice of cement as a bone-void filler. An animal model for vertebroplasty 106
        A clinical trial to assess the feasibility and safety of BAER and VTP for traumatic thoracolumbar fractures . . . 108
        Detailed analysis of intraoperative changes in bone displacement and endplate reduction during balloon
        vertebroplasty visualized with 3D rotational X-ray imaging 110
        A combination of external fixation and balloon vertebroplasty for traumatic fractures 112
    Conclusions 114
Percutaneous kyphoplasty in traumatic fractures (G. Maestretti, S. Krajinovic, and P. Otten) 116
    Terminology 116
    Introduction 116
    History of kyphoplasty 117
    Advantages of percutaneous kyphoplasty 117
    Disadvantages of percutaneous kyphoplasty 117
    Indications for percutaneous kyphoplasty 117
    Contraindications 118
    Surgical technique 118
        Kyphoplasty technique in traumatic fractures 118
        Calcium phosphate cement 120
    Postoperative care 123
    Results of our study 124
        Complications 124
    Critical evaluation 125

Chapter 11. Alternative methods to kyphoplasty: vertebroplasty – lordoplasty (P. F. Heini and R. Orler) 129

Patient evaluation 129
Radiological evaluation 129
Indications and contraindications of vertebroplasty 129
    Contraindications 130
Surgical techniques and augmentation strategies 130
    Materials needed for performance of the operation 130
    Anesthesiological aspects 131
    Screening/imaging 131
    Placing the cannulae 132
    Preparation and injection of the cement 132
Strategies of the augmentation 135

Correction of kyphosis: indication, technique, results 135
Combined surgical procedures 139
Limitations and complications 139

Chapter 12. Injectable cements for vertebroplasty and kyphoplasty (M. Bohner) 143
Various cements 143
Cement properties for vertebroplasty 145
Conclusions 147

Chapter 13. Physiotherapeutic treatment after balloon kyphoplasty – aspects and concepts (Silke Becker) 149
Relation between kyphosis, the diaphragm and breathing 150
Relation between the abdominal wall and pelvic floor muscles, and the deep muscular stabilization system 151
How kyphosis and imbalance of the muscles are related 151
Training and bone density 152
Sensomotoric training 152
Postoperative concepts with sensomotoric training 153
    aerostep® 153
    Mini-trampoline 155
    Outdoor training 156
Kyphosis and incontinence 158

Appendix 161
International coding of diseases according to ICD 10-GM 2004 161
    Coding for osteoporosis 161
    Coding for tumors 161
    Coding for trauma 161
Reimbursement codes per country 161
    Austria 161
    Belgium 162
    France 162
    Germany 162
    Greece 163
    Italy 163
    Netherlands 163
    Ontario 163
    South Africa 164
    Spain 164
    Switzerland 164
    Turkey 164
    UK 164
    USA 165

Contributors

Prof. Dr. Ing. Gamal Baroud
Laboratoire de Biomécanique, Département de génie mécanique, Faculté de génie, Université de Sherbrooke, 2500 boul. de l'Université, Sherbrooke, Québec, Kanada J1K 2R1

Silke Becker, Bsc Physiotherapie
Wirbelsäulenzentrum, 3. Orthopädische Abteilung, Orthopädisches Spital Speising, Speisingerstraße 109, 1130 Wien, Austria

Dr. med. Stephan Becker
Wirbelsäulenzentrum, 3. Orthopädische Abteilung, Orthopädisches Spital Speising, Speisingerstraße 109, 1130 Wien, Austria

PD Dr. med. Ulrich Berlemann
Das Rückenzentrum Thun, Bahnhofstrasse 3, 3600 Thun, Switzerland

Dr. med. Michael Bierschneider
Berufsgenossenschaftliche Unfallklinik Murnau, Prof.-Küntscher-Straße 8, 82418 Murnau, Germany

Prof. Dr. Sc. Tech. Mark Bohner
Head Bone Substitute Materials, Dr. Robert Mathys Stiftung, Bischmattstrasse 12, 2544 Bettlach, Switzerland

Dr. med. Bronek Boszczyk
Orthopädische Universitätsklinik, Inselspital, 3010 Bern, Switzerland

Dr. med. Alexandra Boszczyk
79 Parkside, NG8 2NQ Nottingham, United Kingdom, spinegraphics@gmx.net

Wouter J. A. Dhert
Department of Orthopaedics, University Medical Center Utrecht, Heidelberglaan 100, 3584 CX, Utrecht, The Netherlands

Priv.-Doz. Dr. med. Paul F. Heini
Orthopädische Universitätsklinik, Inselspital, 3010 Bern, Switzerland

Paul A. Hulme, M.Sc.
M. E. Müller Institute for Surgical Technology and Biomechanics, Stauffacherstrasse 78, 3014 Bern, Switzerland

Dr. Hans Jaksche
Berufsgenossenschaftliche Unfallklinik Murnau, Prof.-Küntscher-Straße 8, 82418 Murnau, Germany

Stipe Krajinovic
Medecin assistant clinique de orthopedie, Hopital Catonale de Fribourg, Suisse

Gianluca Maestretti
Medecin adjoint clinique de orthopedie responsable du rachis, Hopital Catonale de Fribourg, Suisse

Dr. Christian Muschitz
Ludwig Boltzmann Institut für Altersforschung, II. Medizinische Abteilung, KH Barmherzige Schwestern, Stumpergasse 13, 1060 Wien, Austria

Univ.-Doz. Dr. med. Michael Ogon
Wirbelsäulenzentrum, 3. Orthopädische Abteilung, Orthopädisches Spital Speising, Speisingerstraße 109, 1130 Wien, Austria

F. Cumhur Oner
Department of Orthopaedics, University Medical Center Utrecht, Heidelberglaan 100, 3584 CX, Utrecht, The Netherlands

Dr. med. Rene Orler
Orthopädische Universitätsklinik, Inselspital, 3010 Bern, Switzerland

Philippe Otten
Medecin agrée neurochirurgien, Hopital Catonale de Fribourg, Suisse

Univ.-Prof. Dr. Heinrich Resch
Ludwig Boltzmann Institut für Altersforschung, II. Medizinische Abteilung, KH Barmherzige Schwestern, Stumpergasse 13, 1060 Wien, Austria

Alexandra Schleyer
Laboratoire de Biomécanique, Département de génie mécanique, Faculté de génie, Université de Sherbrooke, 2500 boul. de l'Université, Sherbrooke, Québec, Kanada J1K 2R1

Dr. med. Othmar Schwarzenbach
Das Rückenzentrum Thun, Bahnhofstrasse 3, 3600 Thun, Switzerland

Jorrit-Jan Verlaan
Department of Orthopaedics, University Medical Center Utrecht, Heidelberglaan 100, 3584 CX, Utrecht, The Netherlands

Sebastian Wolf
Institut für Mechanik und Thermodynamik, Fakultät für Maschinenbau, Chemnitz, University of Technology, 09107 Chemnitz, Sachsen, Germany

Acknowledgement

The editors thank Dr. med. Alexandra Boszczyk for the wonderful illustrations in this book as well as Brigitte Casteels, Vice President International Health Policy & Government Relations, Kyphon International for her support in gathering and analysing reimbursement data.

Furthermore the editors thank all contributing authors for their perseverance and enthusiasm in realising this book.

Chapter 1

Epidemiology of osteoporosis

S. Becker and M. Ogon

During the past decade the number of people affected by osteoporosis has become more significant worldwide, and this disease is now regarded by the WHO as one of the ten most serious global diseases. The aging of the population will probably be one of the most important changes in society throughout the next decades. The incidence of fractures as a consequence of osteoporosis increases exponentially with age [Felsenberg 2002], with the spine being the most common place for osteoporotic fractures [Dennison 2002]. Studies in the USA show indications of vertebral fractures in 25% of women over the age of 75 and in more than 50% of women over 80. The area most frequently affected is the middle range of the thoracic spine and the transition area between the thoracic and lumbar spines [Melton 1989; Kanis 1992; Lee 1996].

In 1998 the European Commission for Employment and Social Affairs developed a consensus paper that reflects the state of osteoporosis at that time in the countries of the EU [European Commission 1998]. In general, osteoporosis is a disease of old age, and therefore the growth of the population within the EU should be analyzed in order to estimate the risk and the further epidemiological development. As is well known, the populations of industrial nations are increasingly aging, and the European Commission of Health has taken up the case and analyzed the problem. The analysis shows that the population of the EU (without the states that joined in 2004) will increase to approx. 390 million people by 2015, and then will go down as a result of the declining birth-rate, falling to approx. 170 million women and 163 million men by 2050. At the same time the ratio of working-age persons to retired persons will change; in particular, the proportion of retired people over the age of 80, that is the population with the highest sex-independent osteoporosis risk, will rise from 8.9 million women and 4.5 million men in 1995 to 26.4 million women and 17.4 million men in 2050 as a consequence of the overall aging of the population. This means a tripling of this elderly age group. In urbanized countries the proportion of persons over the age of 80 will be 5–10% of the general population.

Incidence and prevalence of vertebral fractures

Every year 700,000 Americans and 490,000 EU citizens (EU before 2004) suffer an osteoporotic vertebral fracture [Riggs 1995; O'Neill 1996]. In 1993 the incidence in women over 50 was 18 per 1000 person years [Melton 1993], and thus at that time was already twice as high as the incidence of fractures of the femur neck (6.2 per 1000 person years). Furthermore, only every third osteoporotic fracture is diagnosed correctly and only 10% of the fractures need hospital treatment [Cooper 1992]. According to a study from the UK only every tenth fracture is diagnosed correctly [Van Staa 2001]. Even if a fracture does show on the x-ray, it is not always identified by the diagnosing radiologist and thus will not appear in the patient's file [Gehlbach 2000].

Further data show that the risk for white women over 50 suffering a spontaneous osteoporotic vertebral fracture in their further life is 40% [Riggs 1995; Melton 1989, 1992]. Approximately 8% of all women who are treated with vitamin D and calcium suffer an osteoporotic vertebral fracture within one year after starting treatment [Lindsay 2004]. Among patients who have already suffered a spontaneous fracture, 20% are expected to suffer a second fracture within one year [Lindsay 2001]. In principle all patients with osteoporosis are at risk, particularly if they have already suffered one fracture. In this case, the risk of suffering another fracture in another part of the body is 50–100% [Klotzbücher 2000; Wu 2002].

The prevalence of osteoporosis, i.e. the number of people suffering from osteoporosis at a given time, will probably rise within the EU from 23.7 million in 2000 to 37.3 million in 2050, which means an increase of 57% [European Commission 1998]. Until 2020 men will form the larger fraction of the retired population but by 2050 the ratio will change in favor of women. Accordingly, the proportion of the population at high risk for osteoporosis, i.e. women of pensionable age, will increase considerably, which explains the predicted increase in prevalence. Analysis of the progression of prevalence of vertebral fractures in the first ten years after starting vitamin D and calcium treatment shows a prevalence of 33% after five years and 55% after ten years in women without previous fractures. That is, half of the women treated without bisphosphonates suffer an osteoporotic fracture within the first ten years of treatment, and of those women 11% suffer secondary or further vertebral fractures within the first five years and 29% within the first ten years [Lindsay 2004].

Sex differences

Without doubt the danger of acquiring osteoporosis and thus the risk of osteoporotic fractures increases with advancing age. In general, women are regarded as the high-risk group, although exact figures that compare epidemiological data on the spine are missing and available data on men are mainly poor and inconsistent [Harvey 2004]. However, the incidence in men is only 1.9 times lower than in women [Melton 1993], and the European Vertebral Osteoporosis Study (EVOS) found a higher prevalence of kyphotic deformity in men aged 50–64 than in women of the same age [EVOS 1998]. After the age of 65, women show a higher prevalence for pathological kyphosis than men [O'Neill 1996]. Thus it can be stated that osteoporosis is a problem not only affecting women.

Socio-economic consequences

The aging of the population in industrial nations has far reaching socio-economic consequences [Barrett-Connor 1995; Lippuner 1997]. In 1998 the above mentioned commission divided the then EU countries into three groups, according to their ratio of "working population versus pensioners," indicating the burden on the respective health systems [European Commission 1998]. High-risk countries are those where it is expected that the ratio of work-

ing population to pensioners will increase by 157–171% within the next decade. Germany is at the top of the list of the high risk-group, followed by Ireland, Luxemburg, the Netherlands and Spain. These countries will probably have to increase their gross national product (GNP) by more that 2% in order to keep up with the increasing costs within their health systems. The best ratio of working population to pensioners, with an increase of 85–121%, is expected in Belgium, Denmark, France, Sweden and Great Britain. According to the judgment of the EU Commission these countries might be able to deal with the increasing costs for health services with a GNP increase of 1–1.5% by redistributing resources. All other countries that were members of the EU before 2004 and not mentioned here lie between these two groups.

The demographic development of industrialized countries, and this surely applies worldwide, shows the challenge that health systems are facing in order to accommodate the costs of the diseases of old age. As an example, take Germany, the country with the largest national economy in the EU. A study in 1998 showed an osteoporotic fracture incidence for Germany and the EU [EVOS 1998] as follows:

- 4.1 million people in the EU (2.2 million women /1.9 million men) suffered from an old or acute vertebral fracture in 1998. Another 6.4 million people (4.8 million women/1.6 million men) over the age of 50 were at risk of suffering a fracture. Every year more than 74,000 suffer a new vertebral fracture, i.e.
- 204 vertebral fractures occur every day, 9 vertebral fractures every hour, and one new vertebral fracture happens every 7 minutes [Felsenberg 2002].

A prospective study shows the following results for 2002 for vertebral fractures in the EU (155 million women and men between 50 and 79):

- 1.4 million vertebral fractures every year, 3835 each day, 160 per hour, and 3 fractures per minute [EPOS – European Prospective Osteoporosis Study, Felsenberg 2002].

The costs for immediate therapy were predicted to be 150 million euros for 2001 in Germany, and the resulting costs (e.g. after a fracture) to amount to 5 billion euros. As a comparison: treatment costs for cardio-vascular diseases for the same year were 2.3 million euro, and 700 million for rheumatism. It is also interesting to compare the costs of vertebral fractures with the costs of femoral neck fractures. On average, 150,000 femoral neck fractures occur every year, mostly caused by osteoporosis, and the yearly cost of treatment alone is 3.3 billion euros. The costs incurred can be easily related to these fractures, because they require clinical treatment. Thus in 2002 [Dennison 2002], with an estimated 450,000 new osteoporotic vertebral fractures per year, costs of 340 million euros were predicted for the entire EU, and 13 billion dollars for the USA [Riggs 1995]. As already shown, the data do not reflect the high proportion of unrecorded cases, and thus treatment costs are difficult to estimate and are surely considerably higher. Costs arising in the future are certain to be immense, with the 80-year-olds alone doubling in number. Faced with this fact the EU has implemented programs to inform about osteoporosis, the means of its prevention and the possibilities of treatment.

References

Barrett-Connor E (1995) The economic and human costs of osteoporotic fracture. Am J Med 98(2A): 3–8

Cooper C, Atkinson EJ, O'Fallon WM, Melton LJ 3rd (1992) Incidence of clinically diagnosed vertebral fractures: a population-based study in Rochester, Minnesota, 1985–1989. J Bone Miner Res 7(2): 221–7

Dennison E, Cooper C (2002) Epidemiology of osteoporotic fractures. Horm Res 54 [Suppl] 1: 58–63

European Commission. Directorate-General for Employment, Industrial Relations and Social Affairs. Directorate V/F.2. Report on osteoporosis in the European Community 1998. Luxembourg: Office for Official Publications of the European Communities. ISBN 92-828-5333-0

EVOS (1998) Europäische Studie zur vertebralen Osteoporose – Ergebnisse aus den deutschen Studienzentren. Med Klin 93 [Suppl II]: 3–66

Felsenberg D, Silman AJ, Lunt M, et al (2002) For the European Prospective Osteoporosis Study (EPOS) Group. Incidence of vertebral fracture in Europe: results from the European Prospective Osteoporosis Study (EPOS). J Bone Miner Res 17: 716–24

Felsenberg D, Wieland E, Hammermeister Ch, Armbrecht G, Gowin W, Raspe H; EVOS Gruppe in Deutschland (1998) Prävalenz der vertebralen Wirbelkörperdeformationen bei Frauen und Männern in Deutschland. Med Klin 93 [Suppl II]: 31–4

Gehlbach SH, Bigelow C, Heimisdottir M, May S, Walker M, Kirkwood JR (2000) Recognition of vertebral fracture in a clinical setting. Osteoporos Int 11(7): 577–82

Harvey N, Cooper C (2004) Epidemiology of vertebral fractures. Adv Osteoporotic Fract Manag 3(3): 78–83

Kanis JA, Pitt FA (1992) Epidemiology of osteoporosis. Bone 13 [Suppl 1]: S7–15

Lee YL, Yip KM (1996) The osteoporotic spine. Clin Orthop (323): 91–7

Klotzbuecher CM, Ross PD, Landsman PB, Abbott TA 3rd, Berger M (2000) Patients with prior fractures have an increased risk of future fractures: a summary of the literature and statistical synthesis. J Bone Miner Res 15(4): 721–39

Lindsay R, Pack S, Li Z (2004) Longitudinal progression of fracture prevalence through a populationof postmenopausal women with osteoporosis. Osteoporos Int

Lindsay R, Silverman SL, Cooper C, Hanley DA, Barton I, Broy SB, Licata A, Benhamou L, Geusens P, Flowers K, Stracke H, Seeman E (2001) Risk of new vertebral fracture in the year following a fracture. JAMA 285(3): 320–3

Lippuner K, von Overbeck J, Perrelet R, Bosshard H, Jaeger P (1997) Incidence and direct medical costs of hospitalizations due to osteoporotic fractures in Switzerland. Osteoporos Int 7(5): 414–25

Melton LJ 3rd, Chrischilles EA, Cooper C, Lane AW, Riggs BL (1992) Perspective. How many women have osteoporosis? J Bone Miner Res 7(9): 1005–10

Melton LJ 3rd, Kan SH, Frye MA, Wahner HW, O Fallon WM, Riggs BL (1989) Epidemiology of vertebral fractures in women. Am J Epidemiol 129(5): 1000–11

Melton LJ 3rd, Lane AW, Cooper C, Eastell R, O'Fallon WM, Riggs BL (1993) Prevalence and incidence of vertebral deformities. Osteoporos Int 3(3): 113–9

O'Neill TW, Felsenberg D, Varlow J, Cooper C, Kanis JA, Silman AJ (1996) The prevalence of vertebral deformity in european men and women: the European Vertebral Osteoporosis Study. J Bone Miner Res 11(7): 1010–8

Riggs BL, Melton LJ 3rd (1995) The worldwide problem of osteoporosis: insights afforded by epidemiology. Bone 17 [Suppl 5]: 505–11

van Staa TP, Dennison EM, Leufkens HG, Cooper C (2001) Epidemiology of fractures in England and Wales. Bone 29(6): 517–22

Wu F, Mason B, Horne A, Ames R, Clearwater J, Liu M, Evans MC, Gamble GD, Reid IR (2002) Fractures between the ages of 20 and 50 years increase women's risk of subsequent fractures. Arch Intern Med 162(1): 33–6

Chapter 2

Drug therapy of osteoporosis

H. Resch and C. Muschitz

Drug therapy of osteoporosis is fundamentally changing. Treatments that are available today can halve the risk of a vertebral fracture within months. These drugs are effective at the cellular level, either by inhibiting the resorption of bone via direct or indirect effects on osteoclasts, or, as in the case of teriparatide, by the almost exclusive induction of osteoblasts. The latest development is stable strontium, the salt of ranelic acid. Strontium ranelate is the first drug that simultaneously increases osteogenesis and decreases bone resorption. Recombinant monoclonal antibodies that influence the regulation of osteoclasts at the cytokine level are also currently being developed. Thus in future, in addition to the two present categories of osteotrophic substances (absorption-inhibiting and bone-increasing compounds), there will be two new categories: dual-acting bone agents (DABAs) and cytokines or biologicals.

The range of drugs that are currently available for postmenopausal osteoporosis [Dimai 2002] include several bisphosphonates, one selective estrogen receptor modulator (Raloxifen), teriparatid, fhPTH (1–34), a recombinant form of native parathyrin, various calcitonins (salmon calcitonin, elcatonin), fluorides (sodium fluoride, disodium monofluorophosphate) and strontium ranelate. Following the most recent discussions about possible side-effects of conjugated estrogens and estrogen derivatives, either with or without gestagen, there remain very few selective diagnostic indications that call for hormone treatment of osteoporosis. Evidence-based medicine shows that bisphosphonates, Raloxifen, parathormone and strontium ranelate clearly reduce the risk of a vertebral fracture. Calcitonin and substitution of estrogens or hormones show weaker evidence of reducing the risk of a vertebral fracture. Alendronate, risedronate and strontium ranelate also show strengths in reducing the risk of femoral neck fractures. Vitamin D and calcium formulas, individual or in combination, are available for adjuvant therapy, which, in cases of calcium and/or vitamin D deficiency, also have the ability to influence the risk of a fracture. The preference for a specific drug ultimately depends on the patient's sex and age, his or her fracture risk profile, the bone density values, and possibly existing contraindications.

Pathogenic mechanism and pharmacological effects

Regardless of etiological factors, all forms of osteoporosis result from disorder of bone remodeling; that is, the permanent process of renewal of adult bone, marked by a linked increase and decrease of matrix, is irregular. Permanent osteogenesis is vital, as non-dynamic bone loses its biomechanical quality. Up to one million basic multicellular units (BMU) are active at every moment in the adult skeleton. In each of those units a process unfolds, starting with the osteoclast-induced absorption of bone, followed by formation of new osteoblast bone matrix, and finally two phases of mineralization of the newly synthesized matrix [Parfitt 1979]. These actions are controlled at a higher level by hormones and by mechanical stimulation and physical stress on the bone [Klaushofer 1996]. A number of cytokines and other regulatory proteins are locally effective. The maturation and activation of osteoclasts is influenced by proinflammatory cytokines and by the RANK/RANK ligand/osteoprotegerin system [Hofbauer 2004]. Whereas Raloxifen and antiresorptives of the bisphosphonate family operate at a cellular level on the overactive osteoclast, on the one hand leading to apoptosis but on the other hand regulating the differentiation and precursors of osteoclasts, monoclonal RANKL-antibodies are regarded as one of the most potent regulation inhibitors of the neogenesis of osteoclasts, and also lead to the inhibition of exuberant bone resorption [Lacey 1998]. Osteoblasts are mainly generated and differentiated by the so-called bone morphogenetic protein (BMP). Pharmacotherapeutically this is where bone anabolics such as fluorides, but also teriparatides, are effective. The resting bone marrow cell is regarded as the key progenitor cell from which the active osteoblast develops under the influence of teriparatides.

Therapeutic goals

The terms prevention and therapy of osteoporosis should be differentiated [Marcus 2002]. The prevention of postmenopausal osteoporosis is understood as the application of bone-effective drugs in order to stop further loss of bone mass, provided that osteoporosis, by definition, is not present. The treatment of postmenopausal osteoporosis is understood as the application of bone-effective therapeutics in order to prevent first or further fractures when, according at least to the densitometric criteria, an osteoporotic fracture seems likely. The term secondary prevention is understood as the application of bone-specific substances in patients who already suffer from osteoporotic fractures, in order to prevent further fractures.

Overall there are four treatment goals to be achieved, which are listed below in order of clinical importance for the patient.

1) The treatment of pain

Modern analgesics particularly and opioides in all galenic forms have a quick and, for the patient, tangible effect; transcutaneous applications have the highest patient compliance, thus enabling rapid mobilization. The limiting adverse effects of the past have lost importance as a result of the good prospects of controlling the dosage and to modern Galenism. Currently a widely established analgesic effect is proven only for (salmon) calcitonin, which can be explained by a centrally operating component, among others [Lyritis 1999; Yoshimura 2000]. The often postulated analgesic effect of bisphosphonates is somewhat speculative and has not been convincingly proven [Rovetta 2000].

2) Reduction of the risk of fracture

Fractures after inadequate or minimal trauma present the complication of osteoporosis. Typical locations of fractures associated with osteoporosis are the thoracic and lumbar vertebral bodies, the distal radius and the femoral neck. Moreover, every osteoporotic fracture increases the risk of another fracture five- to seven-fold [Klotzbuecher 2000; Khan 2001]. Thus, the main aim of osteoporosis treatment is, also in the sense of secondary prevention, to achieve lasting reduction of the fracture risk. There is now well documented evidence that some substances can halve the risk of vertebral fracture within months. Nevertheless, the influence of extraskeletal factors that can lead to reduction of the fracture risk independently of pharmacotherapy should also be considered [Valtola 2002; Frost 2001].

3) Increase of bone density

An increase of bone density within osteoprotective treatment is usually associated with reduction of the fracture risk. The extent to which the fracture risk changes in relation to the increase of bone density can vary according to the drug used [Wasnich 2000; Cummings 2001, 2002; Hochberg 1999; Meunier 2004]. Drugs that both increase the bone density and also lead to distinct reduction of absorption markers seem to be effective in reducing non-vertebral fractures.

Nonetheless, bone density changes as the sole criterion for the effectiveness of an osteoprotective therapy are of limited use in identifying a definitive effect on the fracture risk, as they do not indicate biomechanical changes or changes of the material properties of the osseous tissue.

4) Influencing biochemical markers of bone metabolism

Biochemical markers of bone turnover contain markers of ossification (e.g. alkaline phosphatase, osteocalcin, PICP type I procollagen) as well as of osteoclastic activity (cross-links, ICTP, collagen telopeptides). The diagnostic value of such markers is doubtful: thus far no direct links to bone mineral density or fracture risk have been proven [Marcus 1999; Looker 2000]. However, these markers are widely used as a monitoring method to verify the effectiveness of a treatment, especially in studies with larger populations, [Miller 1999], although unfortunately they do not provide evidence on the individual therapeutic response. The fact that laboratory assays for bone metabolism markers have not yet been standardized should also be taken into account. In antiresorptive treatments, reduction of resorption markers seems to be associated with increase of bone density and reduction of the fracture risk [Meunier 2004]. Drugs with an osteoanabolic

Drug therapy of osteoporosis

Table 1. Indications for a drug therapy for osteoporosis (if a combination of findings listed in the columns 1, 2, and 3 applies, and after ruling out secondary osteoporosis and differential diagnoses)

Results	Plus additional results	Plus DXA T-score
Postmenopausal woman/old man	Vertebral fracture (verified by x-ray)	< –2
	Minimal traumatic peripheral fracture (radius, humerus, femoral neck, or tibia)	< –2.5
	Underweight (BMI < 20)	
	High risk of falling (2 or more incidents of domestic falling within the last 6 months	
Begin of a chronic glucocorticoid therapy (> 7.5 mg prednisolone equivalent > 6 months) or fractures with glucocorticoid therapy (independent of dose and duration)	Detection of a vertebral fracture	< –1.5 < –1.0
Chronic glucocorticoid therapy for more than 6 months (> 7.5 mg prednisolone equivalent)	Detection of a vertebral fracture	< –2.5 < –1
High risk of a secondary osteoporosis		Depending on the basic disease

effect lead to an increase of both absorption markers and formation markers, resulting in an increase of bone density and reduction of the fracture risk [Finkelstein 1994; Neer 2001].

Indication for osteoporosis therapy

According to the WHO, the indication for osteoporosis therapy is based on the T-Score, which is determined from the measurement of bone density and defines four diagnostic categories: normal, osteopenia, osteoporosis, and severe (or manifest) osteoporosis. These categories are defined by the deviation of the bone mineral density, which is measured by dual X-ray absorptiometry, from the mean normal value of young adults with healthy bones. The extent of the deviation (in standard deviation) is expressed as the T-Score. Thus postmenopausal women may be classified according to these categories by densitometry with the DEXA method and with an accurate fracture history. Each of the four categories is linked to a recommendation on how to proceed (therapeutically), enabling decisions for further management [Kanis 1994]. For example, if a patient belongs to the category "osteoporosis", the appropriate treatment should be given, whereas the category "normal" is linked to the recommendation

"no therapy is necessary". This algorithm helps with decisions to a certain extent but fails in cases where, in spite of a normal bone mineral density, a fracture occurs after minimal trauma. Postmenopausal women already showing one or more risk factors for an osteoporotic fracture in addition to suffering from extreme osteopenia are also not taken into account [Black 2001]. In the light of recent epidemiological findings, it would therefore make sense to adjust the original scheme and begin treatment when the conditions showing in Tables 1 and 2 apply [American Association of Clinical Endocrinologists 2001].

Treatment options

Basic medication with calcium-vitamin D

Calcium

The adult skeleton contains an average of 1000–1300 g calcium and loses 250–300 mg every day as the result of the transformation activities of bone and to excretion [Mundy 1999]. In consequence, this amount of dietary calcium is needed every day for well balanced calcium homeostasis. As the transintestinal absorption of calcium lies at around 30%, accordingly more calcium should be taken. In the postmenopause, the daily loss of calcium and the

Table 2. Bone mineral density values and fracture risk

Diagnostic category	T score (DEXA)	Fracture risk	Consequence
Normal BMD	> –1.0	Low	No intervention
Osteopenie	–1.0 to –2.5	Medium	a) prevention especially with perimenopausal women b) state the dynamics of bone loss c) treatment especially of older patients with "fragility fracture"
Osteoporosis	< –2.5	High	a) for younger patients: eliminate triggering or enhancing factors b) full anti-osteoporotic therapy especially with patients < 75a
Manifest osteoporosis	< –2.5 + 1-e or several "fragile fractures"	Very high	a) eliminate of triggering/enhancing causes b) full anti-osteoporotic therapy strongly indicated

demand for new calcium for the skeleton is greater, as the result of the increased process of bone absorption [Rodriguez-Martinez 2002].

The daily calcium requirement for a postmenopausal woman is approximately 1000–1200 mg. The daily calcium dose should be based on the average supply of calcium with the food, bearing in mind that some components of food, e.g. oxalic acid (spinach, rhubarb) or phytic acid (bran, wholemeal products), can lead to non-absorbable calcium complexes. There is some evidence that in women adequate calcium substitution can reduce both the postmenopausal loss of bone density and the risk of vertebral fracture [Cummings 1997] [Dawson-Hughes 1990; Recker 1996; Reid 1995]. In addition, it is proven that the effect of adequate calcium supplementation on bone mineral density is most distinct within the first year of therapy [Mackerras 1997].

The possibility of overdosage with resulting hypercalcemia is unlikely, because of the intestinal absorption mechanisms for calcium, and can be expected only when the daily dose is higher than 2500 mg [The North American Menopause Society 2001]. The question of developing kidney stones as a consequence of calcium intake has not yet been clearly answered, but daily doses of up to 1500 mg could possibly lead to reduction of the same.

The combination of calcium with vitamin D

The combination of adequate doses of calcium and vitamin D has proven to make sense in both prevention and treatment of postmenopausal osteoporosis. The positive effect on the skeleton seems to result mainly from the additive effect of calcium and vitamin D, as well as from reduction of the concentration of serum parathormone [Dawson-Hughes 1997], which usually increases with age. In older postmenopausal women with vitamin D deficiency, combining daily doses of 1200 mg calcium with 800 I.E. (20 µg) vitamin D appears to reduce the risk of femoral-neck and other non-vertebral fractures [Chapuy 1992, 1994].

In prospective, randomized, placebo-controlled studies with very small numbers of postmenopausal women, treatment with active vitamin D (Calcitriol) and corresponding correction of the daily calcium supply showed significant effect on the bone mineral density and the fracture risk [Aloia 1988; Gallagher 1990].

Hormone replacement therapy – a fundamental change in evaluation

Recent literature provides much undisputed evidence for the positive effect of hormone replacement therapy (HRT) on bone metabolism and fracture rates. Nevertheless, ongoing discussions about the benefits and risks of conjugated estrogens and estrogen derivatives, with or without gestagen, for the prevention of postmenopausal osteoporosis suggest that such treatments should be used only in carefully chosen indications and should be monitored very closely. There are only very few selective diagnostic indications that call for HRT.

All clinical studies have shown that HRT leads to an increase of bone mass, and recent prospective data prove beyond question that the incidence of vertebral and non-vertebral fractures is reduced [Rossouw 2002]. Further advantages of HRT are improved quality of life and reduction of the incidence of colon cancer. On the other hand there is heated debate about increased cardio- and cerebrovascular and venous thromboembolic incidents [Cauley 2003], though the risks of myocardial infarction and breast cancer have been relativized and even revised in meta-analytic studies. The benefits and risks of HRT for osteological indications should therefore be weighed individually; especially since in the last five years large treatment studies have revealed other, non-endocrine, treatment options to increase bone mass and reduce the risk of fracture. It is without doubt that HRT can be used for prevention of osteoporosis in postmenopausal women who have a high fracture risk and show an incompatibility to other drugs approved for the prevention of osteoporosis, or for whom those drugs are contraindicated.

Substances that inhibit bone absorption

Bisphosphonates

Bisphosphonates are analogs of pyrophosphates, which were described for the first time in the 1960s. Their effect is based on the inhibition of bone absorption, which is achieved both directly by acting on the osteoclasts and indirectly by primarily affecting the osteoblasts. Bisphosphonates are currently the gold standard in treatment of osteoporosis. Treatment studies on the effects on bone mass and risk reduction of vertebral and peripheral fractures are considered as therapy directives and every new drug has to be compared with the results of these large studies before it can take its place among the other treatments. Peroral and parenteral drugs (Clodronat, pamidronate, ibandronate, zoledronate) are currently approved and registered for treatment of postmenopausal osteoporosis as the peroral form alendronate and risedronate.

Older women are at high risk of vertebral and peripheral fractures and are the group for whom oral bisphosphonates are indicated. In numerous clinical studies investigating clinical relevance, alendronate and risedronate have shown similar reduction of the risk of vertebral (35–50%) and non-vertebral (35–50%) fractures [Cranney 2002; Reginster 2000]. The effects are detectable after only six months. Although the oral and increasingly the parenteral bisphosphonates are common therapy options, there still are no standardized guidelines for optimum length of treatment. Data show that ten years' alendronate [Bone 2004] and eight years' risedronate therapy [Sorensen 2003] lead to a lasting increase in bone density, but as our knowledge of bone structure increases, concerns about long-term suppression of bone restructuring arise. The question of whether long-term increase of bone mineralization encourages the development of microfissures remains unanswered [Mashiba 2000]. Once-weekly dosages are now available for both alendronate (70 mg) and risedronate (35 mg) [Schnitzer 2000; Brown 2002], which make daily peroral dosages of bisphosphonates a less appealing alternative, even though studies with comparable fracture data are still missing. Parenteral bisphosphonates gain importance in the case of undesirable gastrointestinal side effects of oral treatments, or where patients have limited compliance and/or disturbed gastrointestinal absorption [Recker 2004], they have been recently approved for treatment of osteoporosis (e.g. ibandronate, zoledronate) [Rosen 2001].

Ibandronate is a highly potent aminobisphosphonate of the third and latest generation. Ibandronate is extremely well tolerated and, because of its particular structure, allows low but highly efficient dosing with prolonged intervals. Approval for treatment of osteoporosis is based on the results of a fracture study examining oral use, with both continuous and intermittent regimens. The incidence of further vertebral fractures was reduced by 62% with the continuous regimen and by 50% with the intermittent regimen. The incidence of non-vertebral fractures was reduced by 69% in a selected high-risk group. In a continuing non-inferiority study it was shown that monthly doses of 50 mg/50 mg on two consecutive days have the same effects on bone density and bone metabolism as a single dose of 100 mg or 150 mg, and are better than a daily continuing regimen with 2.5 mg [Recker et al. 2004a]. Parenteral intravenous doses of 2 mg/2 months and 3 mg/3 months as bolus injection was also examined in a second non-inferiority study [Recker et al. 2004b]. Ibandronate is approved as Bonviva for treatment of osteoporosis and as Bondronat for treatment of skeletal metastasis after breast cancer.

Selective estrogen-receptor modulators

Raloxifen is a selective estrogenic receptor modulator (SERM) that has either an estrogen-agonistic or an estrogen-antagonistic effect, depending on the tissue: it has the former effect on bone and on lipid metabolism, and the latter effect on endometrium and breast tissue [Mitlak 1999]. The effectiveness of the drug in significantly reducing the risk of vertebral fracture in postmenopausal women has been clearly proven [Ettinger 1999] and is always accompanied by an increase of the lumbar bone density [Cummings 2002]. Reduction of the risk of femoral-neck fracture has not yet been demonstrated. In addition to the effect on bone tissue, a 76% reduction of breast cancer risk and a 90% reduction of an estrogenic-receptor-positive breast cancer risk were shown within the same study population. Furthermore, significant reduction of cardiovascular risk was shown in women who already had an increased risk for cardiovascular disease [Barrett-Connor 2002]. However, although there is good gastrointestinal compliance, there is a slight risk for venous thromboembolic events.

Calcitonins

A salmon calcitonin spray for intranasal use (Salm-Calcitonin), salmon calcitonin for sub-cutaneous administration (Salm-Calcitonin), and a synthetic eel calcitonin derivative are currently available on the market. The recommended daily dose for the nasal spray is 200 IU, and positive effects on bone density and risk of vertebral fracture were achieved with a continuous daily dosage at this level [Chestnut 2000]. Under these conditions, the effect on bone density can still be proven after five years of use. Reduction of the risk of femoral neck fracture has not yet been convincingly proven.

Tibolone

Tibolone is a synthetic steroid that shows estrogenic, progestagenic and, to a certain extent, androgenic effects. In some countries, this steroid is also registered as a drug for the prevention of postmenopausal osteoporosis. The positive effect of tibolone on bone is primarily due to stimulation of estrogenic receptors [Kloosterboer 2001]. A daily dose of 1.25 mg or 2.5 mg tibolone appears to increase the bone mineral density of the axial skeleton, lower arm and femoral neck [Berning 1996; Gallagher 2001], probably as a result of inhibition of bone absorption [Bjarnason 1997]. The question of whether tibolone can also lower the fracture risk cannot be answered at present, as no significant studies are available.

Substances that increase bone formation

Parathormone

With the development and registration of teriparatide (rhPTH) [1–34] and rhPTH [1–84], an indisputably effective bone anabolic treatment for advanced osteoporosis is available, the first since the introduction of fluorides. Teriparatide is a recombinant form of native parathormone (PTH) and consists of the first 34 N-terminal amino-acids [Dobnig 1997].

Unlike the historic fluoride therapy, it is now possible for the first time not only to change bone mineralization but also to influence bone structure in a positive way. This mechanism of action clearly differs from that of bisphosphonates, which mainly reduce bone metabolism and increase the mean mineralization of the bone matrix but do not lead to an increase of actual bone mass. The primary target cell for PTH is the osteoblast, where the hormone is bound by type I PTH/PTHRP receptors and triggers several effects by activating a signal transduction mechanism [Schmidt 1995]. This is followed by stimulation of the production of various growth factors such as IGF-1, IGF-2 and TGF-β [Rubin 2002]. One of the first cellular effects, which can be found after only a few days of intermittent PTH use, is the transformation of resting bone parietal cells into active osteoblasts [Dobnig 1995]. The drug is applied subcutaneously by means of injection pens. According to the available data, duration of treatment is limited to 18 months and must be followed by an antiresorptive therapy if the newly gained bone mass is to be preserved. At the end of the largest treatment study to date [Neer 2001], the bone density of the spine had increased by 9.7% (compared with 1.1% in the placebo group) and of the femoral neck by 2.8% (compared with –0.7% in the placebo group). The rate of new vertebral fractures was reduced by 65%, the rate of multiple vertebral fractures by 73%. The number of non-vertebral fractures was too small to allow any conclusions about the effectiveness of the drug on the various fracture locations.

Combination therapies

The effects of a combination of antiresorptive drugs have been examined in only a few prospective randomized studies. Combined or consecutive administration of antiresorptive and anabolic drugs has not yet been examined in any adequate studies. No data are available on a possible influence on the fracture risk.

Parathormone and antiresorptives

For a long time the prevailing opinion was that inhibition of bone absorption with simultaneous stimulation of bone formation should have a better effect than the respective mono-therapies. Two recent publications, however, do not verify this hypothesis. The use of PTH on its own produced a greater increase in lumbar bone density than monotherapy with alendronate or a combination of the two drugs [Schmidt 1995; Rubin 2002]. If absorption-inhibiting drugs are given after PTH treatment, preservation and even further increase of bone density can be shown, whereas the gain in bone density is slowly lost if anti-absorptive treatment is not given [Finkelstein 2003; Black 2003].

Fluorides

The effect of fluorides on bone is mediated through stimulation of osteoblast differentiation and proliferation [Farley 1983]. In particular, the trabecular bones not only react with an increase of bone density in dependence on the dose [Riggs 1990, 1994; Pak 1995] but also show dysmorphic changes of the micro-architecture, which can be verified radiologically and histologically [Fratzl 1994; Kleerekoper 1996]. Whether this seemingly inconsistent effect is due to the dose, the type of fluoride used, or to Galenism, or a combination of these factors, cannot yet be answered with any certainty [Haguenauer 2000]. Nevertheless, the optimum therapeutic range is probably 20–30 mg of available fluorides daily. A concluding judgement on the effect of sodium fluoride on fracture risk is not yet possible. The weight of undisputed data on other therapeutic agents and their beneficial effect on bone density and reduction of fracture risk means that, at present, fluoride treatment has lost its importance.

Substances with a synchronous effect on bone formation and absorption

Strontium ranelate (SR) is the first substance that simultaneously increases bone regeneration and decreases bone absorption, leading to positive physiological balance of bone metabolism and distinctly better bone quality.

In vitro, SR increases the replication of pre-osteoblastic cells, leading to an increase in genesis of collagen and in synthesis of bone matrix proteins [Boivin 1996]. At the same time, inhibition of osteoclast differentiation and a direct inhibiting effect on these cells lead to reduction of bone absorption. In clinical studies in postmenopausal women [Meunier 2002, 2004], SR lowered the relative risk of vertebral fracture (44% yearly) in addition to increasing the bone density (7.3%). In the TROPOS study [Reginster, 2004] of more than 5000 women, SR achieved significant reduction (16%) in the relative risk for one or more non-vertebral fractures ($p < 0.05$), compared with the placebo. In addition, there was a 41% reduction of fracture risk of the hip joint ($p < 0.025$) within the first 18 months of the study. The increase in bone density of the femoral neck was significantly greater in the SR group and showed a relative change of 6.54% in comparison with the placebo group ($p < 0.001$). The serum level of bone-specific alkaline phosphatase (BALP) also increased in the SR group, whereas NTx in the urine decreased. This provides further confirmation of the broad effect of SR. Furthermore, this drug has proven to be very well tolerated; the daily dose is 2 g and treatment should continue for three years. At present there are no known significant side effects.

Substances with a biological effect

The RANKL antibody – new approaches in the treatment of osteoporosis

The discovery of the receptor-activator of the nuclear factor-κB ligand (RANKL) from the TNF superfamily has led to a better understanding of the cell biology of osteoclasts. RANKL leads to activation of RANK, which is also found on the osteoclast cell in its preliminary stages. This mechanism encourages not only the formation and activation of osteoclasts but also their survival by suppressing apoptosis [Hsu 1999]. RANKL itself is in turn expressed by osteoblasts in order to maintain osteoporotic homeostasis. The secretory glycoprotein osteoprotegerin (OPG) is the natural antagonist of RANKL and its activity is also controlled by cytokines and hormones [Simonet 1997]. Disturbances of this balance inevitably lead to the development of bone diseases as a result of increased bone absorption.

Monoclonal antibody Denosumab offers a new approach in the treatment of osteoporosis and other diseases accompanied by increased bone absorption; for example, multiple myeloma or bone metastasis in breast and prostate cancers. Experiments with inactivated RANKL in mice demonstrated artificially induced osteoporosis resulting from the maintained function of osteoblasts, which in turn resulted from the non-activation of osteoclasts [Kong 1999]. AMG 162 antibody binds to RANKL and thus blocks the fusion and activation of RANK.

The first dose-determining study in postmenopausal women was published in early 2004 and demonstrated a placebo-controlled and, depending on the dose, rapid reaction (within 12 hours), as well as sustaining a constant reduction (up to six months) in serum and urine bone-specific markers (NTx) after a single subcutaneous injection [Bekker 2004]. The bone-formation marker BALP, the intact PTH and the serum-calcium level did not change during the treatment, apart from initial variation. This can be seen as a demonstration of the antiresorptive potency of Denosumab. The injection was tolerated well by all the patients; not one showed significant changes in serum chemistry or in T or B lymphocytes. Nine months after the injection the antibodies could no longer be traced chemically.

Following the above study, the first double-blind, placebo-controlled phase III study with approximately 7000 untreated women with manifest osteoporosis was carried out in late 2004.

Osteoporosis in men

Prevention and therapy

The principles for prevention of fractures are similar for both men and women; it is essential to minimize the risk factors. Attention should be paid to smoking habits, insufficient intake of calcium and/or vitamin D, excessive consumption of alcohol and insufficient exercise. Current guidelines recommend 1200 mg calcium and 400–600 IU vitamin D daily after the age of 50 [Dawson-Hughes 1997].

Few studies have dealt specifically with the treatment of men suffering from osteoporosis. In the first major study testing a bisphosphonate over a period of two years in men suffering from osteoporosis, alendronate achieved significant increase of bone density in both the lumbar and hip areas irrespective of testosterone and estradiol levels in the serum. In addition, there was a decrease of vertebral fractures during the study period [Kurland 2000].

It was also observed in men suffering from osteoporosis caused by glucocorticoids that both alendronate and risedronate showed positive effects on bone density and reduced the incidence of vertebral fractures.

PTH treatment, which has already shown excellent increases of bone density and reduction of the fracture incidence in postmenopausal women with osteoporosis, also seems to have huge potential in osteoporosis treatment in men [Orwoll 2000].

References

Aloia JF, Vaswani A, Yeh JK, Ellis K, Yasumura S, Cohn S (1988) Calcitriol in the treatment of postmenopausal osteoporosis. Am J Med 84: 401–8

American Association of Clinical Endocrinologists (2001) Medical guidelines for clinical practice for the prevention and management of postmenopausal osteoporosis. Endocrine Pract 4(7): 294–312

Barrett-Connor E, Grady D, Sashegyi A, Anderson PW, Cox DA, Hoszowski K, Rautaharju P, Harper KD (2002) Raloxifene and cardiovascular events in osteoporotic postmenopausal women. JAMA 287(7): 847–57

Bekker P, Holloway D, Rasmussen A, Murphy R, Martin S, Leese P, Holmes G, Dunstan C, DePaoli A (2004) A single-dose-controled study af AMG 162, a fully human monoclonal antibody to RANKL, in postmenopausal women. J Bone Miner Res 19: 1059–66

Berning B, Kuijk CV, Kuiper JW, Bennink HJ, Kicovic PM, Fauser BC (1996) Effects of two doses of tibolone on trabecular and cortical bone loss in early postmenopausal women: a two-year randomized, placebo-controlled study. Bone 19(4): 395–9

Bjarnason NH, Bjarnason K, Hassager C, Christiansen C (1997) The response in spinal bone mass to tibolone treatment is related to bone turnover in elderly women. Bone 20(2): 151–5

Black DM, Greenspan SL, Ensrud KE, Palermo L, McGowan JA, Lang TF, Garnero P, et al (2003) The effects of parathyroid hormone and alendronate alone or in combination in postmenopausal osteoporosis. N Engl J Med 349: 1207–15

Black DM, Steinbuch M, Palermo L, Dargent-Molina P, Lindsay R, Hoseyni MS, Johnell O (2001) An assessment tool for predicting fracture risk in postmenopausal women. Osteoporos Int 12: 519–28

Boivin G, Deloffre P, Perrat B, Panczer G, Boudeulle M, Mauras Y, Allain P, Tsouderos Y, Meunier PJ (1996) Strontium distribution and interactions with bone mineral in monkey Iliac bone after Strontium Salt (S12911) Administration. J Bone Miner Res 11(9): 1302–11

Bone HG, Hosking D, Devogelaer JP, Tucci JR, Emkey RD, Tonino RP, Rodriguez-Portales JA, Downs RW, Gupta J, Santora AC, Liberman UA (2004) Ten years experience with alendronate for osteoporosis in postmenopausal women. N Engl J Med 350: 1189–99

Brown JP, Kendler DL, McCLung MR, Emkey RD, Adachi JD, Bolognese MA, Li Z, Balske A, Lindsay R (2002) The efficacy and tolerability of risedronate once a week for the treatment of postmenopausal osteoporosis. Calcif Tissue Int 71: 103–11

Cauley JA, Robbins J, Chen Z, Cummings SR, Jackson RD, LaCroix AZ, Le Boff M; Women's Health Initiative Investigators, et al (2003) Women's Health Initiative Investigators: effects of estrogen plus progestin on risk of fracture and bone mineral density: the Women's Health Initiative randomized trial. JAMA 290: 1729–38

Chapuy MC, Arlot ME, Delmas PD, Meunier PJ (1994) Effect of calcium and cholecalciferol treatment for three years on hip fractures in elderly women. BMJ 308: 1081–2

Chapuy MC, Arlot ME, Duboeuf F, Brun J, Crouzet B, Arnaud S, Delmas PD, Meunier PJ (1992) Vitamin D3 and calcium to prevent hip fractures in elderly women. N Engl J Med 327: 1637–42

Chesnut CH III, Silverman S, Andriano K, et al (2000) (PROOF Study Group). A randomized trial of nasal spry salmon calcitonin in postmenopausal women with established osteoporosis: the Prevent Recurrence of Osteoporotic Fractures Study. Am J Med 109: 267–76

Chestnut CH, Skag A, Christiansen C, et al (2004) Effects of oral ibandronate administered daily or intermittently on fracture risk in postmenopausal osteoporosis. J Bone Miner Res 19: 1241–9

Cranney A, Wells G, Willan A, Griffith L, Zytaruk N, Robinson V, Black D, et al (2002) Meta-analysis of alendronate for the treatment of postmenopausal women. Endocr Rev 23: 508–16

Cumming RG, Nevitt MC (1997) Calcium for prevention of osteoporotic fractures in postmenopausal women. J Bone Miner Res 12: 1321–29

Cummings SR, Karpf DB, Harris F, Genant HK, Ensrud K, LaCroix AZ, Black DM (2002) Improvement in spine bone density and reduction in risk of vertebral fractures during treatment with antiresorptive drugs. Am J Med 112: 281–9

Cummings SR (2001) The paradox of small changes in bone density and reductions in risk of fracture with raloxifene. Ann N Y Acad Sci 949: 198–201

Dawson-Hughes B, Dallal GE, Krall EA, Sadowski L, Sahyoun N, Tannenbaum SA (1990) A controlled trial of the effect of calcium supplementation on bone density in postmenopausal women. N Engl J Med 323: 878–83

Dawson-Hughes B, Harris SS, Krall EA, Dalla GE (1997) Effect of calcium and vitamin D supplementation on bone density in men and women 65 years of age or older. NEJM 337: 670–6

Dimai HP, Pietschmann P, Resch H, Klaushofer K (2002) Leitfaden zur medikamentösen Therapie der postmenopausalen Osteoporose. Für die EBM-Arbeitsgruppe der Österr. Ges. zur Erforschung des Knochens und Mineralstoffwechsels (AuSBMR). Wien Med Wochenschr 152 (23–24): 596

Dobnig H, Turner RT (1995) Evidence that intermittent treatment with parathyroid hormone increases bone formation in adult rats by activation of bone lining cells. Endocrinology 136: 3632–8

Dobnig H, Turner RT (1997) The effects of programmed administration of human parathyroid hormone fragment (1–34) on bone histomorphometry and serum chemistry in rats. Endocrinology 138: 4607–12

Ettinger B, Black DM, Mitlak BH, Knickerbocker RK, Nickelsen T, Genant HK, Christiansen C, Delmas PD, Zanchetta JR, Stakkestad J, Glueer CC, Krueger K, Cohen FJ, Eckert S, Ensrud K, Avioli LV, Lips P, Cummings SR (1999) Reduction of vertebral fracture risk in postmenopausal women with osteoporosis treated with raloxifene: results from a 3-year randomized clinical trial. JAMA 282: 637–45

Farley JR, Tarbaux N, Baylink DJ (1983) Fluoride directly stimulates proliferation and alkaline phosphatase activity of bone-forming cells. Science 222: 330–2

Finkelstein JS, Hayes A, Hunzelman JL, Wyland JJ, Lee H, Neer RM, et al (2003) The effects of parathyroid hormone, alendronate, or both in men with osteoporosis. N Engl J Med 349: 1216–26

Finkelstein JS, Klibanski A, Schaefer EH, Hornstein MD, Schiff I, Neer RM (1994) Parathyroid hormone for the prevention of bone loss induced by estrogen deficiency. N Engl J Med 331(24): 1618–23

Fratzl P, Roschger P, Eschberger J, Abendroth B, Klaushofer K (1994) Abnormal bone mineralization after fluoride treatment in osteoporosis: a small-angle x-ray scattering study. J Bone Miner Res 9(10): 1541–9

Frost HM (2001) Should future risk-of-fracture analyses include another major risk factor? The case for falls. J Clin Densitom 4(4): 381–3

Gallagher JC, Baylink DJ, Freeman R, McClung M (2001) Prevention of bone loss with tibolone in postmenopausal women: results of two randomized, double-blind, placebo-controlled, dose-finding studies. J Clin Endocrinol Metab 86(10): 4717–26

Gallagher JC, Goldgar D (1990) Treatment of postmenopausal osteoporosis with high doses of synthetic calcitriol. Ann Int Med 113: 649–55

Haguenauer D, Welch V, Shea B, Tugwell P, Adachi JD, Wells G (2000) Fluoride for the treatment of postmenopausal osteoporotic fractures: a meta analysis. Osteoporos Int 11: 727–38

Hochberg MC, Greenspan S, Wasnich RD, Miller P, Thompson DE, Ross PD (2002) Changes in bone density and turnover explain the reduction in incidence of non-vertebral fractures that occur during treatment with antiresorptive agents. J Clin Endocrinol Metab 87(4): 1586–92

Hochberg MC, Ross PD, Black D, Cummings SR, Genant HK, Nevitt MC, Barrett-Connor E, Musliner T, Thompson D (1999) Larger increases in bone mineral density during alendronate are associated with a lower risk of new vertebral fractures in women with postmenopausal osteoporosis. Fracture Intervention Trial Research Group. Arthritis Rheum 42(6): 1246–54

Hofbauer LC, Kuhne CA, Viereck V (2004) The OPG/RANKL/RANK system in metabolic bone diseases. J Musculoskelet Neuronal Interact 4(3): 268–75

Hsu H, Lacey DL, Dunstan CR, et al (1999) Tumor necrosis factor receptor family member RANK mediates osteoclast differentiation and activation induced by osteoprotegerin ligand. Proc Natl Acad Sci USA 96: 3540–5

Kanis JA, WHO Study Group (1994) Assessment of fracture risk and its application to screening for postmenopausal osteoporosis: synopsis of a WHO report. Osteoporos Int 4: 368–81

Khan SA, de Geus C, Holroyd B, Russel AS (2001) Osteoporosis follow-up after wrist fractures following minor trauma. Arch Intern Med 161: 1309–12

Klaushofer K, Peterlik M (1996) Pathophysiology of osteoporosis. In: Bröll H, Dambacher MA (eds) Osteoporosis: a guide to diagnosis and treatment. Karger, Basel

Kleerekoper M (1996) Fluoride and the skeleton. Crit Rev Clin Lab Sci 33(2): 139–61

Kloosterboer HJ (2001) Tibolone: a steroid with a tissue-specific mode of action. Steroid Biochem Mol Biol 76: 231–8

Klotzbuecher CM, Ross PD, Landsman PB, Abbot TA III, Berger M (2000) Patients with prior fractures have an increased risk of future fractures: a summary of the literature and statistical synthesis. J Bone Miner Res 15: 721–39

Kong YY, Yoshida H, Sarosi I, Tan HL, Timms E, Capparelli C, Morony S, Oliveira-dos SA, Van G, Khoo W, Wakeham A, Dunstan CR, LAcey DL, Mak TW, Boyle WJ, Penninger JM (1999) OPGL is a key regulator of osteoclastogenesis, lymphocyte development and lymph node organogenesis. Nature 397: 315–23

Kurland ES, Cosman F, McMahon DJ, Rosen CJ, Lindsay R, Bilezikian JP, et al (2000) Parathyroid hormone as a therapy for idiopathic osteoporosis in men: effects on bone mineral density and bone markers. J Clin Endocrinol Metab 85: 3069–76

Lacey DL, et al (1998) Osteoprotegerin (OPG) ligand is a cytokine that regulates osteoclast differentiation and activation. Cell 93: 165–76

Looker AC, Bauer DC, Chesnut III CH, Gundberg CM, Hochberg MC, Klee G, Kleerekoper M, Watts NB, Bell NH (2000) Clinical use of biochemical markers of bone remodeling: current status and future directions. Osteoporos Int 11: 467–80

Lyritis GP, Ioannidis GV, Karachalios T, Roidis N, Kataxaki E, Papaiannou N, Kaloudis J, Galanos A (1999) Analgesic effect of salmon calcitonin suppositories in patients with acute pain due to recent osteoporotic vertebral crush fractures: a prospective double-blind, randomized, placebo-controlled clinical study. Clin J Pain 15(4): 284–9

Mackerras D, Lumley T (1997) First- and second-year effects in trials of calcium supplementation on the loss of bone density in postmenopausal women. Bone 21(6): 527–33

Marcus R, Holloway L, Wells B, Greendale G, James MK, Wasilauskas C, Keleghan J (1999) The relationship of biochemical markers of bone turnover to bone density changes in postmenopausal women: results from the Postmenopausal Estrogen/Progestin Interventions (PEPI) trial. J Bone Miner Res 14: 1583–95

Marcus R, Wong Mayme, Heath H, Stock JL (2002) Antiresorptive treatment of postmenopausal osteoporosis: comparison of study designs and outcomes in large clinical trials with fracture as an endpoint. Endocr Rev 23: 16–37

Mashiba T, Hirano T, Turner CH, Forwood MR, Johnston CC, Burr DB (2000) Suppressed bone turnover by bisphosphonates increases microdamage accumulation and reduces some biomechanical properties in dog rib. J Bone Miner Res 15: 613–20

Meunier PJ, Roux C, Seemann E, Ortalani S, et al (2004) The effects of strontium ranelate on the risk of vertebral fracture on women with postmenopausal osteoporosis. N Engl J Med 350: 459–68

Meunier PJ, Slosman DO, Delmas PD, et al (2002) Strontium ranelate: Dose dependent effects in established postmenopausal vertebral osteoporosis – A 2 year randomized placebo controlled trial. J Clin Endocrinal Metab 87: 2060–6

Miller PD, Barran DT, Bilezikian JT (1999) Practical clinical applications of biochemical markers of bone turnover: consensus of an expert panel. J Clin Densitom 2: 323–42

Mitlak BH, Cohen FJ (1999) Selective estrogen receptor modulators: a look ahead. Drugs 57: 653–63

Mundy GR, Guise TA (1999) Hormonal control of calcium homeostasis. Clin Chem 45(8): 1347–52

Neer RM, Arnaud CD, Zanchetta JR, Prince R, Gaich GA, Reginster JY, Hodsman AB, Eriksen EF, Ish-Shalom S, Genant HK, Wang O, Mitlak BH (2001) Effect of parathyroid hormone (1–34) on fractures and bone mineral density in postmenopausal women with osteoporosis. N Engl J Med 344(19): 1434–41

Orwoll E, Ettinger M, Weiss, et al (2000) Alendronate for the treatment of osteoporosis in men. N Engl J Med 343: 604–10

Pak CYC, Sakhaee K, Adams-Huet B, Piziak V, Peterson RD, Poindexter JR (1995) Treatment of postmenopausal osteoporosis with slow-release sodium fluoride. Ann Int Med 123: 401–8

Parfitt AM (1979) Quantum concept of bone remodelling and turnover: implications for the pathogenesis of osteoporosis. Calcif Tissue Int 28: 1–5

Recker RR, Hinders S, Davis KM, Heaney RP, Stegman MR (1996) Correcting calcium nutritional deficiency prevents spine fractures in elderly women. J Bone Miner Res 11: 1961–6

Recker RR, Kendler DL, Adami S, Hughes C, Dumont E, Schimmer RC, Cooper C (2004a) Monthly oral ibandronate significantly reduces bone resorption in postmenopausal osteoporosis: 1-year results from MOBILE. Poster SA406, presented at: 26th Annual Meeting of the American Society for Bone Mineral Research, October 1–5, Seattle, WA

Recker RR, Reid DM, Sambrook, P, Hughes C, Ward P, Bonvoisin B, Adami S (2004b) Intermittent intravenous ibandronate injection regimens provide at least equivalent efficacy to daily Oral Ibandronate: 1-year results from DIVA. Arthritis Rheum 50 [Suppl]: S513

Reginster J, Minne HW, Sorensen OH, Hooper M, Roux C, Brandi ML, Lund B, Ethgen D, Pack S, Roumagnac I, Eastell R (2000) Randomized trial of the effects of risedronate on vertebral fractures in women with established postmenopausal osteoporosis. Vertebral Efficacy with Risedronate Therapy (VERT) Study Group. Osteoporos Int 11: 83–91

Reginster J-Y, Sawicki A, Devogelaer JP, et al (2004) Stontium ranelate reduces the risk of hip fracture in women with postmenopausal osteoporosis. Oral presentation, 26th Annual Meeting of the ASBMR. Seattle, Abstract 855

Reid IR, Ames RW, Evans MC, Gamble GD, Sharpe SJ (1995) Long-term effects of calcium supplementation on bone loss and fractures in postmenopausal women: a randomized controlled trial. Am J Med 98(4): 331–5

Riggs BL, Hodgson SF, O'Fallon WM, Chao EY, Wahner HW, Muhs JM, Cedel SL, Melton LJ III (1990) Effect of fluoride treatment on the fracture rate in postmenopausal women with osteoporosis. N Engl J Med 322: 802–9

Riggs BL, O'Fallon WM, Lane A, Hodgson SF, Wahner HW, Muhs J, Chao E, Melton LJ III (1994) Clinical trial of fluoride therapy in postmenopausal osteoporotic women: extended observations and additional analysis. J Bone Miner Res 9(2): 265–75

Rodriguez-Martinez MA, Garcia-Cohen EC (2002) Role of Calcium and vitamin D in the prevention and treatment of osteoporosis. Pharmacol Ther 93: 37–49

Rosen LS, Gorden D, Kamisnki M, et al (2001) Zoledronat acid versus pamidronate in the treatment of skeletal metastases in patients with breast cancer or osteolytic lesions of multiple myeloma: a phase III, double-blind, comparative trial. Cancer J 7: 377–87

Rossouw JE, Anderson GL, Prentice RL, LaCroix AZ, Kooperberg C, Stefanick ML, Jackson RD, et al (2002) Risks and benefits of estrogen plus progestin in healthy postmenopausal women: principal results from the Women's Health Initiative randomized controlled trial. JAMA 288: 321–33

Rovetta G, Monteforte P, Balestra V (2000) Intravenous clodronate for acute pain induced by osteoporotic vertebral fracture. Drugs Exp Clin Res 26(1): 25–30

Rubin MR, Cosman F, Lindsay R, Bilezikian JP (2002) The anabolic effects of parathyroid hormone. Osteoporos Int 13: 267–77

Russel RG, Rogers MJ (1999) Bisphosphonates: from the laboratory to the clinic and back again. Bone 25(1): 97–106

Schmidt IU, Dobnig H, Turner RT (1995) Intermittent parathyroid hormone treatment increases osteoblast number, steady state messenger ribonucleic acid levels for osteocalcin, and bone formation in tibial metaphysis of hypophysectomized female rats. Endocrinology 136: 5127–34

Schnitzer T, Bone HG, Cepaldi G (2000) Therapeutic equivalence of alendronate 70 mg once-weekly and alendronate 10 mg daily in the treatment of osteoporosis. Aging 12: 1–12

Simonet, et al (1997) Osteoprotegerin: a novel secreted protein involved in the regulation of bone density. Cell 89: 309–19

Sorensen O, Goemare S, Wenderoth D, Chines A, Roux C (2003) Sustained effect of risedronate: a 7-year study in postmenopausal women. Calcif Tissue Int 72: 402, P-275

The North American Menopause Society (2001) The role of calcium in peri- and postmenopausal women. Consensus opinion of the North American Menopause Society 8: 84–95

Valtola A, Honkanen R, Kroger H, Tuppurainen M, Saarikoski S, Alhava E (2002) Lifestyle and other factors predict ankle fractures in perimenopausal women: a population-based prospective cohort study. Bone 30(1): 238–42

Wasnich RD, Miller PD (2000) Antifracture efficacy of antiresorptive agents are related to changes in bone density. J Clin Endocrinol Metab 85: 231–6

Yoshimura M (2000) Analgesic mechanism of calcitonin. J Bone Miner Metab 18(4): 230–3

Chapter 3

Clinical aspects and mortality risk of the osteoporotic spine fracture

S. Becker and M. Ogon

Clinical diagnosis of spinal fracture

In general, a fracture is clinically diagnosed by localizing the pain; however, this simple clinical feature is not reliable in the case of osteoporotic fractures of the spine, where up to 20% are incidental radiological findings, without the patient consciously experiencing pain [Cooper 1992]. Delayed diagnosis is a further problem. Osteoporotic fractures generally occur spontaneously without a traumatic incident and also partly respond well to analgesics, therefore the radiological diagnosis, if the fracture is diagnosed at all, is often delayed. In addition, many patients never go to a doctor but are treated by physiotherapists or masseurs [Ross 1991]. In contrast, patients with advanced collapse of a vertebral body and a resulting deformity have a higher level of pain and thus are diagnosed sooner and treated earlier than patients with simpler fractures [Watts 1991].

Two groups of patients can be distinguished regarding the course. The first group presents the cases described above, showing a distinctive vertebral collapse accompanied by immediate persisting pain that improves gradually within the following weeks and months. The second group of patients presents only light fractures accompanied by mild pain. However, this group often develops recurrent pain, which can last up to 18 months. Furthermore, this group is characterized by progressive collapse of one or several vertebrae [Lyritis 1989] and by progressive loss of the physiological posture [Ryan 1994]. Several fractures can occur in the same vertebra in this period. This inhomogeneity of symptoms generally leads to delayed diagnosis, so that patients with vertebral fractures are often not treated until four weeks after the onset of pain [Cooper 1992]. With our own patients also, we have observed periods of 4–6 weeks between the pain event and the presentation at our hospital [Becker 2004]. There are many clinical effects of the two courses, which vary from slightly deformed compression fractures and "pseudoarthroses" with persisting instability [McKiernan 2003] (see also chapter on osteonecrosis) to multiple fractures with loss of posture [Heini 2004] and fractures with consecutive neurocompression (Fig. 1).

Neurological failures as a consequence of pure osteoporotic sintering fractures are rare, but can occur [Leech 1990; Heggeness 1993; Korovessis 1994]. Particular cases of complete paralysis are also described [O'Connor 2002].

The pain is often typically located in the area of the fractured vertebra, without any radicular symptoms [Silverman 1992]. The important clinical symptoms become obvious during palpation and percussion, as clinical examination of a fresh osteoporotic fracture is always painful. In our experience, thoracolumbar fractures are not only locally painful but the pain also extends to the lumbosacral transition area. In general, an operation is not indicated if there is no local pain. As is well known, spinal pain can have multiple causes, therefore locally induced pain caused by palpation and percussion is the only reliable clinical sign for an acute osteoporotic fracture of the spine.

The duration of pain varies according to the groups mentioned above; there are reports of pain lasting up to six months [Ringe 1987] and within our own cases we see patients who still have pain in the fracture area up to 12 months later. However, after such a long time, multiple fractures or delayed fracture cure, e.g. after taking cortisone, should always be considered.

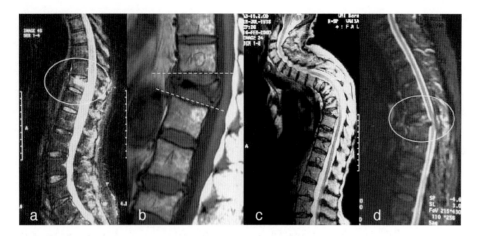

Fig. 1. Spectrum of the spinal problems related to osteoporosis [Radiographs by P. F. Heini, Bern]. **a** Plain vertebral fracture with persisting pain lasting 2 months. **b** Pseudoarthosis of Th 11-6 months after a fracture. The instability causes pain when changing position. **c** Multiple vertebral fractures within the thoracic spine with a consecutive disturbance of equilibrium and severe hyperlordosis of the cervical spine. **d** Th 7 fracture with spinal stenosis and myelon compression; the patient shows signs of gait ataxia

The course of the pain is variously described in the literature, but all authors agree that within the first two weeks after fracture there is no distinct change of pain and no change in consumption of analgesics [Gennari 1991; Lyritis 1990; Montagnini 1989]. Under conservative treatment, significant reduction of pain could not be observed until the third week after osteoporotic fracture; pain reduction of 40% was described after 30 days [Gennari 1991].

The clinical consequences of a spinal fracture

The biomechanical changes after a vertebral fracture and kyphosis are described in Chapter 4. Clinical consequences after a kyphotic deformity lie in a higher risk of recurrent spinal fracture and of secondary fractures in another part of the skeleton.

The risk of recurrent vertebral fracture is on a different aspect. Primarily the risk of subsequent fractures increases with the number of prevalent fractures, ie the more primary vertebral fractures occur, the higher is the risk of a secondary vertebral fracture. The risk increases from 3.2 (relative fracture risk compared with the healthy population) after the first vertebral fracture to 23.3 after the third [Lunt 2003]. Furthermore the risk depends on the type of fracture: an anterior or mid-vertebral fracture has a higher fracture risk (5.9, relative fracture risk compared with the healthy population), whereas a pure posterior fracture has a lower risk of 1.6. The localization of the prevalent fracture also plays a role: the presence of a vertebral deformity at baseline increases the risk of an incident fracture six-fold compared with absence of deformity at baseline, but the risk varies with the distance from the baseline deformity. For example, if the subsequent fracture lies within three vertebral bodies on either side of prevalent fracture, the relative fracture risk is 7.7, compared with a lower risk of 4.0 if the subsequent fracture is more than three healthy vertebral bodies distant from the primary fracture.

These findings from the European Prospective Study on Osteoporosis (EPOS, Lunt 2003) give a clear indication of the necessity of preventing or treating a kyphotic deformity in order to lower the subsequent fracture rate.

The changed posture due to the kyphosis results in a distinctly uncertain gait and increases the risk of falls [Lynn 1997; Skelton 2001]. As a result, in their further history approximately one third of the patients will suffer from one or several peripheral fractures in addition to the spine fracture. Most incidents involve the wrist, then the humerus head; these are followed by fractures of the femur neck and tibia [Vega 1990]. Specific postoperative balance training is therefore essential for these patients, and because of the importance of this topic, we have dedicated a whole chapter to this treatment (see Chapter 12).

The lung is another organ system which immediately causes increased mortality after fractures of the spine. Kyphosis significantly reduces the vital capacity (VC) and the forced expired volume (FEV) [Culham 1994; Di Bari 2004; Schlaich 1998]. Up to 10% reduction of the VC was detected in patients with an osteoporotic spine fracture [Leech 1990; Schlaich 1998]. Reduction of the VC in particular indicates a restrictive lung disease [Schlaich 1998]. Mass screening of patients with chronic obstructive pulmonary disease (COPD) detected a significantly high frequency of osteoporotic fractures of the spine [Papaioannou 2003]. A corresponding reduction of pulmonary function could also be diagnosed in patients with other restrictive lung diseases caused by kyphotic deformity (ankylosing spondylitis, severe kypho-scoliosis etc.) [Kafer 1977; Kroker 1991; Leech 1985]. We know from scoliosis surgery that pulmonary function increases with the straightening of the thorax [Kovac 2001]; this also applies to osteoporotic kyphosis.

Apart from the physical changes, the psyche of the patient is also affected. The changes in physical appearance and posture lead to social isolation and loss of self-esteem, loss of independence and loss of drive [Linnel 1991], and in the end to a loss of quality of life [Cook 1993; Silverman 1992].

Mortality after fractures of the spine (Table 3)

The mortality rate after vertebral fractures is increased as the consequence of accompanying diseases, especially pulmonary changes as described

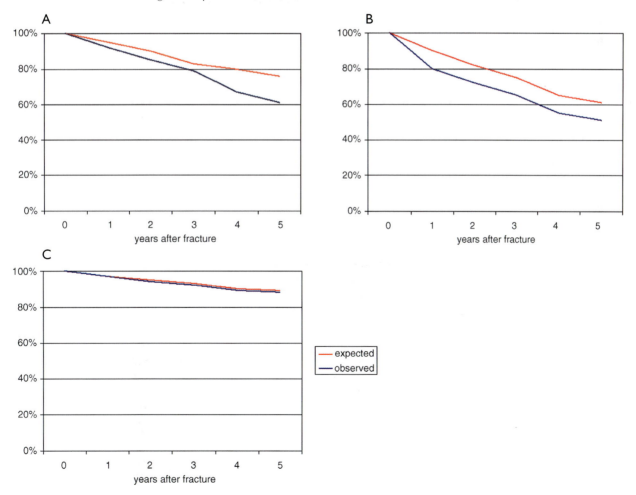

Table 3. **A** Survival rate after osteoporotic vertebral fractures. **B** Survival rate after femur neck fractures. **C** Survival rate after wrist fracture. According to Cooper et al. (1992)

above. Many studies describe increased mortality after spinal fractures [Hasserius 2003; Chesnut 1997; Lyles 1993; Gold 1996; Ismail 1998], and in the five years after a fracture the increase may be up to 23% (15–37%) [Browner 1991; Cooper 1993; Kado 1999]. Increased mortality from lung diseases and lung cancer has also been observed after osteoporotic fractures.

As a result of the kyphosis and accompanying restriction of pulmonary function, patients suffer from lung diseases more frequently after an osteoporotic vertebral fracture and have a mortality risk 2.1 times higher than in healthy people [Kado 1999]. Here the severity of the kyphosis is the crucial point: advanced kyphoses show significant increase of the mortality risk (2.6 times higher than in healthy people [Kado 1999]).

The increased occurrence of lung cancer (1.4-fold increased risk) [Cooper 1993; Kado 1999] can be regarded only as a secondary phenomenon of a paraneoplastic osteoporosis; it seems that these patients already suffer from osteoporosis and an accompanying vertebral fracture before the lung cancer is clinically manifested.

A recent study on the relationship of mortality rate to deformity [Pongchaiyakul 2005] clearly showed a 2.7 times higher mortality rate in patients after vertebral fracture, with the overall highest rate in patients with the lowest bone density and/or kyphotic deformity resulting from a vertebral fracture.

Thus the mortality rate after a spinal fracture is comparable to the mortality rate after a fracture of the femur neck, except that in the latter case the rate is higher in the first six months, whereas the mortality rate after spinal fractures increases in a somewhat linear manner [Cooper 1993]. However, related studies have not taken into account that after a spinal fracture patients have an increased risk of falls because of their changed posture and gait, so the mortality risk is surely higher because of the combination of various injuries.

References

Becker S, Chavanne A, Meissner J, Bretschneider W, Ogon M (2004) Die minimal-invasive chirurgische Versorgung osteoporotischer Wirbelfrakturen mit Vertebroplastie und Kyphoplastie. J Miner Stoffwechs 11 [Sonderheft 1]: 4–7

Browner WS, Seeley DG, Vogt TM, Cummings S (1991) Non-trauma mortality in elderly women with low bone mineral density. Lancet 338: 355–8

Chesnut CH 3rd, Bell NH, Clark GS, Drinkwater BL, English SC, Johnson CC Jr, Notelovitz M, Rosen C, Cain DF, Flessland KA, Mallinak NJ (1997) Hormone replacement therapy in postmenopausal women: urinary N-telopeptide of type I collagen monitors therapeutic effect and predicts response of bone mineral density. Am J Med 102(1): 29–37

Cook DJ, Guyatt GH, Adachi JD, Clifton J, Griffith LE, Epstein RS, Juniper EF (1993) Quality of life issues in women with vertebral fractures due to osteoporosis. Arthritis Rheum 36(6): 750–6

Cooper C, Atkinson EJ, O'Fallon WM, Melton LJ 3rd (1992) Incidence of clinically diagnosed vertebral fractures: a population-based study in Rochester, Minnesota, 1985–1989. J Bone Miner Res 7(2): 221–7

Cooper C, Atkinson EJ, Jacobson SJ, et al (1993) Population-based study of survival after osteoporotic fractures. Am J Epidemiology 137(9): 1001–5

Culham EG, Jimenez HA, King CE (1994) Thoracic kyphosis, rib mobility, and lung volumes in normal women and women with osteoporosis. Spine 19(11): 1250–5

Di Bari M, Chiarlone M, Matteuzzi D, Zacchei S, Pozzi C, Bellia V, Tarantini F, Pini R, Masotti G, Marchionni N (2004) Thoracic kyphosis and ventilatory dysfunction in unselected older persons: an epidemiological study in Dicomano, Italy. J Am Geriatr Soc 52(6): 909–15

Gennari C, Agnusdei D, Camporeale A (1991) Use of calcitonin in the treatment of bone pain associated with osteoporosis. Calcif Tissue Int 49 [Suppl 2]: 9–13

Gold DT (1996) The clinical impact of vertebral fractures: quality of life in women with osteoporosis. Bone 18 [Suppl 3]: 185–9

Hasserius R, Karlsson MK, Nilsson BE, Redlund-Johnell I, Johnell O (2003) Prevalent vertebral deformities predict increased mortality and increased fracture rate in both men and women: a 10-year population-based study of 598 individuals from the Swedish cohort in the European Vertebral Osteoporosis Study. Osteoporos Int 14(1): 61–8

Heggeness MH (1993) Spine fracture with neurological deficit in osteoporosis. Osteoporos Int 3(4): 215–21

Heini PF, Orler R (2004) Vertebroplastie bei schwerer Osteoporose. Technik und Erfahrungen mit multisegmentaler Injektion [Vertebroplasty in severe osteoporosis. Technique and experience with multi-segment injection]. Orthopäde 33(1): 22–30

Ismail AA, O Neill TW, Cooper C, Finn JD, Bhalla AK, Cannata JB, Delmas P, Falch JA, Felsch B, Hoszowski K, Johnell O, Diaz-Lopez JB, Lopez Vaz A, Marchand F, Raspe H, Reid DM, Todd C, Weber K, Woolf A, Reeve J, Silman AJ (1998) Mortality associated with vertebral deformity in men and women: results from the European Prospective Osteoporosis Study (EPOS). Osteoporos Int 8(3): 291–7

Kado DM, Browner WS, Palermo L, et al (1999) Vertebral fractures and mortality on older women. Arch Int Med 159: 1215–20

Kafer ER (1977) Respiratory and cardiovascular function in scoliosis: a review. Bull Eur Physiopath Respir 13: 299–321

Korovessis P, Maraziotis T, Piperos G, Spyropoulos P (1994) Spontaneous burst fracture of the thoracolumbar spine in osteoporosis associated with neurological impairment: a report of seven cases and review of the literature. Eur Spine J 3(5): 286–8

Kovac V, Puljiz A, Smerdelj M, Pecina M (2001) Scoliosis curve correction, thoracic volume changes, and thoracic diameters in scoliotic patients after anterior and after posterior instrumentation. Int Orthop 25(2): 66–9

Kroker PB, Sybrecht GW (1991) Thoraxwanderkrankungen. In: Classen M, Diehl V, Kochsiek E (Hrsg) Innere Medizin. Urban und Schwarzenberg, München, 1: 1157–60

Leech JA, Dulberg C, Kellie S, et al (1990) Relationship of lung function to severity of osteoporosis in women. Am Rev Respir Dis 141: 68–71

Leech JA, Ernst P, Rpgala EJ, et al (1985) Cardiorespiratory status in relation to mild deformity in adolescent idiopathic scoliosis. J Pediatr 106: 143–9

Linnel PW, Hermansen SE, Elias MF, et al (1991) Quality of life in osteoporotic women. J Bone Min Res 6 [Suppl 1] 96: 106

Lunt M, O'Neill TW, Felsenberg D, Reeve J, Kanis JA, Cooper C, Silman AJ; European Prospective Osteoporosis Study Group (2003) Characteristics of a prevalent vertebral deformity predict subsequent vertebral fracture: results from the European Prospective Osteoporosis Study (EPOS). Bone 33(4): 505–13

Lyles KW, Gold DT, Shipp KM, Pieper CF, Martinez S, Mulhausen PL (1993) Association of osteoporotic vertebral compression fractures with impaired functional status. Am J Med 94(6): 595–601

Lynn SG, Sinaki M, Westerlind KC (1997) Balance characteristics of persons with osteoporosis. Arch Phys Med Rehabil 78: 273–7

Lyritis 2 GP, Magiasis B, Eliopoulos A, Tsekoura M, Ioakimidis D (1990) Analgesic effect of salmon calcitonin in cases of osteoporotic vertebral fractures. In: Christiansen C, Overgaard K (eds) Osteoporosis 1990. Osteopress, Copenhagen, pp 1392–5

Lyritis GP, Mayasis B, Tsakalakos N, Lambropoulos A, Gazi S, Karachalios T, Tsekoura M, Yiatzides A (1989) The natural history of the osteoporotic vertebral fracture. Clin Rheumatol 8 [Suppl 2]: 66–9

McKiernan F, Jensen R, Faciszewski T (2003) The dynamic mobility of vertebral compression fractures. J Bone Miner Res 18(1): 24–9

Montagnani M, Gonnelli A, Francini G, Piolini M, Gennari C (1989) Analgesic effect of salmon calcitonin nasal pray on bone pain. In: Mazzuoli GF (ed) Calcitonin 1988 new therapeutic perspectives: the nasal spray. Sandoz AG, Basel, pp 126–33

O'Connor PA, Eustace S, O'Byrne J (2002) Spinal cord injury following osteoporotic vertebral fracture: case report. Spine 27(18): 413–5

Papaioannou A, Parkinson W, Ferko N, Probyn L, Ioannidis G, Jurriaans E, Cox G, Cook RJ, Kumbhare D, Adachi JD (2003) Prevalence of vertebral fractures among patients with chronic obstructive pulmonary disease in Canada. Osteoporos Int 14(11): 913–7

Pongchaiyakul C, Nguyen ND, Jones G, Center JR, Eisman JA, Nguyen TV (2005) Asymptomatic vertebral deformity as a major risk factor for subsequent fractures and mortality: a long-term prospective study. J Bone Miner Res 20(8): 1349–55

Ringe JD (1987) Clinical evaluation of salmon calcitonin in bone pain. In: Christiansen C, Johansen JS, Riis BJ (eds) Osteoporosis 1987. Osteopress, Copenhagen, pp 1262–4

Ross PD, Ettinger B, Davis JW, Melton LJ 3rd, Wasnich RD (1991) Evaluation of adverse health outcomes associated with vertebral fractures. Osteoporos Int 1(3): 134–40

Ryan PJ, Blake G, Herd R, Fogelman I (1994) A clinical profile of back pain and disability in patients with spinal osteoporosis. Bone 15(1): 27–30

Schlaich C, Minne HW, Bruckner T, et al (1998) Reduced pulmonary function in patients with spinal osteoporotic fractures. Osteoporos Int 8: 261–7

Silverman SL (1992) The clinical consequences of vertebral compression fracture. Bone 13 [Suppl 2]: S27–31

Skelton DA (2001) Effects of physical activity on postural stability. Age and Ageing 30(S4): 33–9

Vega E, Mautalen C, Ghiringhelli G, Fromm G (1990) Other sceletal fractures in osteoporotic females with vertebral fractures. In: Christiansen C, Overgaard K (eds) Osteoporosis 1990. Osteopress, Copenhagen, pp 504–6

Watts NB, Genant HK, Harris ST, et al (1991) Clinical correlates of radiographically apparent vertebral fractures. Calcif Tiss 42 [Suppl]: 39

Chapter 4

Biomechanics

Biomechanics of cement injection in vertebroplasty

G. Baroud and A. Schleyer

Summary

Vertebroplasty is being increasingly used for consolidation of osteoporotic vertebrae or other pathological findings; for example, in bone cancer. In this chapter we present a combination of theoretical considerations and *in vivo* and *ex vivo* studies on cement injection. The unexpected results reflect the fact that approximately 95% of the overall injection pressure is necessary for cement delivery through the cannula, and only approximately 5% for the dispersion of cement in the spongiosa. One of our most important findings is that the process of cement injection makes conflicting demands on bone cements, which are required to be more viscous and less viscous at the same time. A low viscosity eases cement delivery through the injection cannula, whereas a high viscosity reduces the risk of cement leakage out of the vertebra. The challenge therefore is to develop biomaterials, techniques and/or devices that can overcome or manage the conflicting demands concerning cement viscosity.

Introduction

Vertebroplasty is a relatively new technique for the treatment of vertebral fractures originating in osteoporosis or resulting from other pathological findings [Cotton et al. 1996; Deramond et al. 1998; Heini et al. 2000; Jensen et al. 1997; Mathis et al. 2001]. In this procedure, bone cement is injected under pressure through a cannula into the porous structure of the cancellous bone. The bone marrow is thereby displaced out of the cavities of the vertebra (Fig. 2). The in situ curing of the cement in these cavities strengthens the weakened vertebra [Heini et al. 2000, 2001; Jensen et al. 1997; Krause et al. 1982;

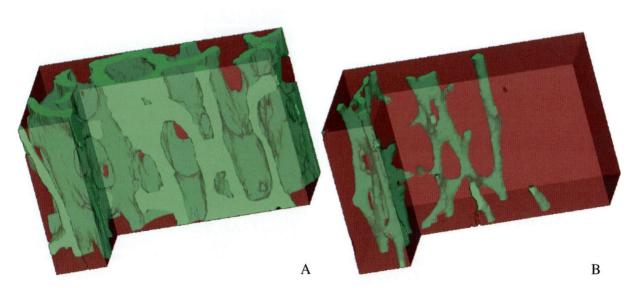

Fig. 2. Pictures of a three-dimensional reconstruction of trabeculae of the spongiosa of healthy (**A**) and osteoporotic bone (**B**). The bone is depicted in turquoise, the bone marrow in violet

Mathis et al. 2001; San Millan Ruiz et al. 1999; Wilson et al. 2000].

Until now it has not been possible to develop uniform standards for the cement-injection procedure. Furthermore, there are no clear guidelines from which to choose the parameters necessary for ensuring reproducible and safe injection with a predictable outcome. Because of this situation, the outcome of cement injection is often unpredictable.

In the following, we present various studies that have contributed to a clearer understanding and therefore to potential enhancements of the injection process.

Initially, we analyzed the process of the injection pressure and injection volume for successful *in vivo* cement injection, an insufficient cement injection (aborted injection because of too high an injection pressure) and a risky *in vivo* injection (aborted because of potential cement leakage out of the vertebra). Because the injection pressure seemed to play an important role in the outcome of an injection, it was further analyzed in a theoretical study. The injection pressure was divided into an extravertebral component (delivery of cement through the cannula) and an intravertebral component (spreading of cement throughout the vertebral cavities). Following the theoretical analysis, the different pressure components were measured and evaluated in an *ex vivo* experiment. We discovered that the major part of the injection pressure is needed for cement delivery.

In addition to examining the injection pressure, we addressed the risk of cement leakage. Specifically, the role of cement rheological properties in cement leakage was examined in both a theoretical and experimental manner.

In the last section of this chapter, we present a newly developed injection cannula, which is expected to significantly reduce the injection pressure. In an additional study, the injection pressures necessary for the new cannula were compared with those for a conventional cannula. For this, *ex vivo* experiments were performed under simulated clinical conditions.

In vivo measurements of injection pressure/volume versus time for three representative cases of vertebroplasty

In this section, the *in vivo* injection data (pressure-versus-time and volume-versus-time) for the three possible outcomes (successful, insufficient, unsafe injection) are described. Details on technique and guidelines for patient selection are described in Heini et al. [2001].

The biomaterial used in all three cases presented here was a low-viscosity acrylic cement (Palacos E-flow, Essex Chemie, Lucerne, Switzerland). Ten milliliters of cement was divided into two 5-cc standard syringes and then injected through a biopsy cannula (8 G, Somatex, Berlin, Germany). After the liquid was added to the powder, there was a waiting period (elapsed time) of approximately 2 minutes, during which time the cement attained the appropriate consistency for safe injection. After this elapsed time, the cement had a handling time of about 3 minutes, during which the procedure had to be completed. The injection data described below (for successful, for insufficient and for risky delivery) are three cases chosen to represent *in vivo* pressure-injection data.

A custom-made sterilizable injection device (Fig. 3) instrumented with force and displacement transducers was used to monitor the injection data and was calibrated using a universal material testing machine (Mini Bionix 856, MTS, Eden Prairie, Minnesota, USA). A 5-cc syringe was filled with cement and placed in the device. The pressure-versus-time and injection volume-versus-time curves of the injection were collected using a Palm Pilot.

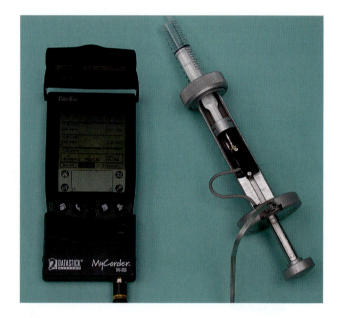

Fig. 3. Device for measuring injection pressure and injection volume. The device consists of a delivery tool, in which you can insert a 5-cc syringe, and a Palm Pilot

On the basis of the cement expansion and the resistance encountered during the first 20 seconds of the injection, the clinician is often able to predict whether or not the injection will be successful. The injection in this case was considered to be successful because the injection forces required were moderate and the cement expansion (infiltration) was uniform.

An injection pressure and volume-versus-time graph is shown in Fig. 4. In this case, two syringes were injected consecutively, with a time delay when the first syringe was replaced by the second. The first syringe was injected over a longer time period than the second syringe because the cement was initially too liquid and thus had to be delivered cautiously. A total of approximately 8.4 cc was injected in strokes of approximately 0.4–1.0 cc. The pressure in response to these strokes varied substantially because of the ongoing cement polymerization. The maximum pressure of the first syringe was approximately 0.5 MPa, for the second one it increased to about 1.7 MPa.

By tactile and visual feedback, the clinician is often able to predict the outcome of the treatment within the first 20 seconds of an injection. The injection is considered successful when the required pressures are moderate and the cement filling in the spongiosa is uniform. An injection is considered insufficient when it is aborted at an early stage because of too high an injection pressure. The injection process in an unsafe injection is aborted at an early stage because the cement leaks; for example, through blood vessels and out of the vertebra, thus endangering the life of the patient.

For the purpose of clarity, only the pressure and volume progression of the successful injection are shown in Fig. 4. Afterwards, they are compared with the results of the insufficient and the unsafe injection. Further results are published in Baroud et al. [2004].

The pressure and volume progression of the insufficient injection showed that, despite a clearly lower injection rate, the injection pressure increased over 2 MPa and therefore the injection had to be aborted. In the case of an unsafe injection, the progression curves were similar to those of the successful injection, therefore presumably factors other than pressure are responsible for cement leakage out of the vertebra.

In summary, it can be concluded that in most cases the injection pressure plays an important role in the outcome of vertebroplasty.

Analysis of injection pressures during vertebroplasty

For a clearer understanding of the pressure mechanisms in vertebroplasty, we divided the overall pressure, which is in equilibration with the injection pressure, into two components: (1) the overall extravertebral injection pressure, which is necessary to overcome the friction between the cement and the cannula wall while delivering cement, and (2) the intravertebral pressure. Equation (I) represents the

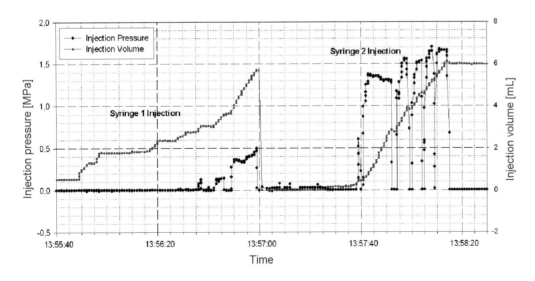

Fig. 4. Injection pressure and injection volume versus time for successful injection

pressure required for the infiltration of cement into the cavities of the spongiosa and for the displacement of bone marrow:

$$P_{inj} = P_{extra} + P_{intra} \qquad (I)$$

where P_{inj} = injection pressure, P_{extra} = extravertebral pressure, and P_{intra} = intravertebral pressure. The intravertebral pressure can be further subdivided into (a) the pressure required to infiltrate the trabecular cavities with cement, and (b) the shell pressure as hydrostatic resistance caused by the displacement of the bone marrow out of the vertebra into the adjacent structure. The hydrostatic resistance strongly depends on the trabecular structure and on the porosity of the vertebral shell. The revised mathematical representation is as follows:

$$P_{inj} = P_{extra} + P_{inf} + P_{komp} \qquad (II)$$

where P_{inf} = infiltration pressure and P_{komp} = shell pressure. To analyze the different components of the injection pressure, we built a theoretical model. The compacta pressure is neglected in this model because it is very complex and there is no way to describe it mathematically. By means of this model, we were able to point out the relationship between the extravertebral pressure and the infiltration pressure, as well as the significance of the physical properties of the cement and the other injection parameters for the injection pressure.

The approach for this model was the equilibrium of the injection force, based on P_{inj}, and the forces evoked by the infiltration pressure P_{inf} and the extravertebral pressure P_{extra} [Baroud et al. 2003]. To describe the infiltration pressure, we used the Law of Darcy (infiltration of a fluid into a porous medium), and for the extravertebral pressure, the Law of Hagen-Poisseuille (flow of a Newtonian fluid through a cylindrical tube):

$$F(P_{inj}) = F(P_{extra}) + F(P_{inf})$$
$$\Rightarrow P_{inj}\pi r_s^2 = P_{inf}\pi r_k^2 + \int_0^l 2\pi\gamma r_k\mu \, dl \qquad (III)$$

where r_s = radius of the syringe, r_k = radius of the cannula, γ = shear rate, μ = cement viscosity, and l = length of the cannula. Because the cement infiltrates the spongiosa uniformly in a successful filling, Darcy's Law can be integrated in spherical coordinates. Assuming that cement flow in the cannula is laminar, the Law of Hagen-Poiseuille can be integrated over the length of the cannula. Accordingly, we can write Eq. (III) for the injection pressure in the following way:

$$\qquad\qquad \text{Summand 1} \qquad\qquad \text{Summand 2}$$
$$\Rightarrow P_{inj} = \mu \frac{Q}{4\pi\kappa} \cdot \left(\frac{1}{r_k} - \frac{1}{r}\right) + \mu \frac{8Q}{\pi r_k^4} l \qquad (IV)$$

where μ = cement viscosity, Q = flow rate, κ = bone permeability, and r = radius of the spreading cement cloud. The first term displays the infiltration pressure P_{inf}, the second term displays the extravertebral pressure P_{extra}. Equation IV shows that the injection pressure depends on a combination of geometrical (e.g., length and radius of a cannula) and physical (e.g., viscosity and flow rate) parameters.

Using values taken from the References [Baroud et al. 2003a, 2004a, b; Krause et al. 1982; Naumann et al. 1999] for μ, Q and κ, as well as the geometrical dimensions of an 8-gauge cannula (l = 200 mm, r_k = 2 mm) in Eq. IV, a very interesting and surprising result emerges: the infiltration pressure of an injection contributes 0% at the beginning and only 5.6% at the end to the overall pressure. Consequently, the extravertebral pressure, which is necessary to overcome the friction in the cannula, has to be considered as the limiting factor for cement injection in vertebroplasty, because it is approximately 95% of the required injection pressure. It is therefore clear that cement delivery through a cannula represents the bottleneck of the cement injection.

Experimental determination of the different pressure components during a cement injection

Using the results of the theoretical consideration of the injection forces, we measured the injection pressure and intravertebral pressure on the lateral shell of the vertebra during an injection process in an *ex vivo* experiment with cadaveric vertebrae. Our assumption, derived from the theoretical model, was that the injection pressure would be much higher than the intravertebral pressure.

For the experiments, 15 lumbar vertebrae were harvested from three osteoporotic spines. The bone mineral density ranged from 0.136 to 0.620 g/cm². The injection cannula with the connected syringe was placed in the vertebra so that it entered the right vertebral pedicle, and its end was placed as accurately as possible one third of the overall width from the right lateral side and one third of the overall length from the frontal side. To measure the intravertebral pressure at the left lateral shell, a pressure sensor was connected to a vent in the compacta of the vertebral body. The overall test arrangement was installed in a servohydraulic-engine test bench, where the integrated load cell measured the injection forces. The schematic test arrangement is shown in Fig. 5. Instead of cement, silicon oil with a comparable viscosity (100 Pa·s) was used, giving reproducible results because of the constant viscosity. More exact information about test preparation and test arrangements can be found in Baroud et al. [2005].

Injection of the silicon oil was carried out under controlled kinematic conditions. The pressure acquired by the load cell that was needed to inject the silicon oil corresponds to the pressure that a physician has to apply manually to a syringe during a vertebroplasty procedure. The intravertebral pressure produced from the cement dispersion in the vertebral body on the lateral shell was acquired with the pressure transducer.

After initiation of the injection process, the injection pressure quickly reached a relatively constant level of (344 ± 62) kPa and did not change significantly during the remainder of the injection process. In contrast to the injection pressure, the intravertebral pressure on the cortical shell increased significantly, though the increase was very slight, with maximal values of (3.54 ± 2.92) kPa. The hypothesis proposed at the beginning of this study was affirmed very clearly, because the measured injection pressure was approximately 97 times higher than the intravertebral pressure.

For a further control, silicon oil was injected into the air, and at the same time, the injection pressure was measured under the same conditions as for the *ex vivo* vertebral body experiments. Comparison of the pressures in both test sequences resulted in nonsignificant differences. This affirms the accuracy/validity of the assumption made at the beginning of the study.

The conclusions drawn from this study are presented in the following. The experiment clearly confirms that the largest amount of the injection pressure is required for cement delivery through the cannula; the intravertebral pressure seems to be minimal. The problem of insufficient filling of a vertebral body resulting from an injection pressure that is too high is not associated with an increase of the intravertebral pressure and is therefore only explainable by a change in the required extravertebral pressure, which has to be regarded as the key factor of the injection process. Methods such as the opening of the shell for release of pressure or making a cavity in the spongiosa do not contribute significantly to reduction in the risk of insufficient filling.

One implication of the findings of our study is that because the shell pressure contributes very little to the overall injection pressure, the shell pressure cannot be important for insufficient cement delivery. However, shell pressure appears to be a significant component of intravertebral pressure, and therefore it is hypothesized that it may be important in how the cement spreads in the vertebral body.

Analysis of risk of cement extravasation out of the vertebral body

In earlier experiments [Baroud et al. 2005; Heini et al. 2000; Jensen et al. 1997; Mathis et al. 2001] it became clear that cement leakage out of the vertebral body (for example, through blood vessels or a fracture line) is a frequently occurring and serious problem in vertebroplasty, and can culminate in nerve damage, pulmonary embolism or even the death of the patient. In this paragraph we consider the influence of various factors on extravasation risk at theoretical and experimental levels.

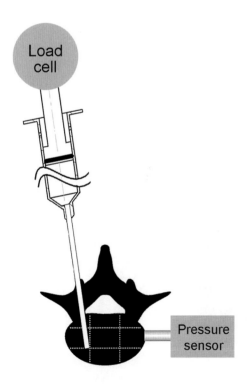

Fig. 5. Schematic representation of the experimental setup for measuring intra- and extravertebral pressure

Because the cement generally chooses the path of least resistance, an "extravasation factor" was analytically calculated in the theoretical model. This factor describes the relation of the pressure necessary for uniform dispersion of the cement and the pressure required for injecting the cement into the leakage path [Bohner et al. 2003]. In addition to the geometrical factors, such as the diameter of the extravasation path or the porosity, which cannot be influenced by the physician and are not further explained here for this reason, the relation of cement viscosity μ_c to the viscosity of bone marrow μ_b plays an important role. From qualitative calculations, we conclude that a low ratio μ_c/μ_b significantly increases the risk of extravasation, whereas increasing the ratio diminishes the risk. For a physician, this means using cement that is as highly viscous as possible. On examining the dependence of cement viscosity on time after mixing the powder with the monomer (μ_c increases with time) [Baroud et al. 2004a], it is possible to increase the cement viscosity while postponing the injection *to* a later point in time. Because of the shear-thinning properties of the cement, it would also be advantageous if one could inject the cement at a low flow rate, which means with a low injection pressure.

Although cement with higher viscosity would reduce the risk of extravasation, there are certain constraints; for example, the trabeculae could break under the too high charge during the injection process, or the delivery system could fail because of the high forces (failing of the syringe), so that there is no longer an optimal connection between bone and cement.

In experiments with a leakage model, we have shown that a higher ratio of cement viscosity to bone marrow viscosity and a delayed injection point reduce the risk of cement leakage. The leakage model consisted of a porous ceramic filter or aluminium foam with porosity similar to that of the spongiosa. The leakage path was simulated by a cylindrical drilling in the test specimen. With the aid of a materials-testing machine, cement was injected through a cannula into the probe. The behavior of dispersion at different moments of the injection after mixing the ingredients became apparent after the injection by means of x-ray images (Fig. 6) of the models and affirmed the theoretical perceptions.

The following problems arose from the results for the injection process. The time scope in which the polymerization process allows an injection is relatively small when injecting cement with a high viscosity. This requires a high flow rate to fill the vertebral body sufficiently and with this, a high injection pressure (Eq. IV). In addition, the injection pressure increases because of the increased cement viscosity. If the injection exceeds the forces a human being can apply, the injection will have to be aborted prematurely. Furthermore, the preferred goal is to have low injection pressures to reduce the extravasation risk as a result of the shear-thinning properties of the cement. The requirements of the injection process for uniform infiltration (high cement viscosity, low pressure) and for sufficient filling of the vertebral bodies are thus exactly *contrary*.

Development of a new injection cannula

On the basis of the results of the preceding studies (the extravertebral pressure represents 95% of the overall injection pressure and is the key factor in the injection process; high viscosity and low pressure are necessary for a uniform dispersion of cement in the spongiosa; low viscosity and high pressure are

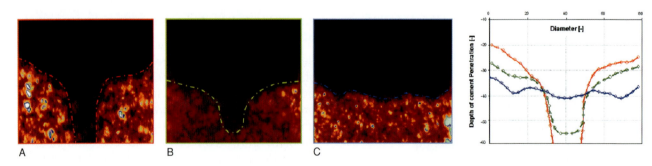

Fig. 6. X-ray pictures of the cement-filling pattern of strong cement leakage (**A**, low-viscous cement), moderate cement leakage (**B**, mid-viscous cement), and no cement leakage (**C**, high-viscous cement). The graph on the right side depicts a digitalization that was made to keep the numeric values for the amount of cement leakage

required for a sufficient filling of the vertebral body), we developed a new injection cannula. The goal of this development was to achieve significant diminution of the extravertebral pressure.

The new injection cannula consists of two parts with different inner and outer diameters (Fig. 7). The distal third of the cannula has the same dimensions as a conventional 8-gauge cannula (inner diameter, 3.38 mm), because this part is introduced through the pediculus arcus vertebrae into the vertebral body and thus has to be adapted to these anatomical conditions. The inner diameter of the proximal part, which partially penetrates the soft tissue, is 6.92 mm, which is nearly double the size of the distal third. The overall length of the new cannula is 135 mm.

A theoretical model, which is based on the law of Hagen-Poiseuille and in which the anthropometry of the human body was incorporated, was established to find the ideal dimensions for the cannula. The result, proven in an earlier experimental study, is that by doubling the inner diameter of the proximal part of the cannula the extravertebral pressure is decreased by 63% compared with a conventional 8-gauge cannula [Baroud and Steffen 2005].

In a further study, the newly developed cannula was tested under simulated clinical conditions. Injection pressures were measured while a surgeon in spinal orthopedics injected bone cement into cadaveric vertebrae through a conventional cannula and through the newly developed cannula under the same injection conditions (e.g., flow and pressure) as in a real vertebroplasty procedure. Details of the experimental setup and accomplishment can be found in Baroud et al. [Baroud et al. 2006]. On the basis of the preceding results, we expected a diminution of the injection pressure of 50–60% with the new cannula.

Altogether, 40 tests per cannula were performed. The ratio of the injection pressures needed to inject the cement through the two cannulas averaged 56%. This means that the new cannula decreases the injection pressure by approximately 44%. A t-test showed that these results have a very high significance ($p < 0.001$). Our hypothesis that the new cannula significantly reduces the injection pressure was proven by the results of this study.

With the lowering of the injection pressure by the new cannula, it is possible to inject more viscous cements without the problem of the required pressures exceeding the forces a surgeon can apply. Thereby, the risk of cement leakage out of the vertebral body and the risk of insufficient filling are reduced. Fortunately, the new cannula is compatible with the standard injection system and is particularly inexpensive.

Conclusions

For a clearer understanding of the injection process in vertebroplasty, analysis of the meaning of injection pressure and cement viscosity was important mainly for the outcome of a treatment.

Consideration of the theoretical model delivered surprising results. Approximately 95% of the overall injection pressure is needed to overcome the friction between the cannula and cement (extravertebral pressure), and only 5% of the overall injection pressure is necessary in the spongiosa (intravertebral pressure). The subsequent results proved that the intravertebral pressure is significantly lower than the extravertebral pressure.

Analysis of the extravasation risk showed that by using more viscous cement the risk can be reduced significantly. Furthermore, a lower injection pressure and a resulting lower intravertebral pressure would be advantageous for the regular spreading of the cement.

To enhance the injection process, we have developed a new cannula that through its geometry

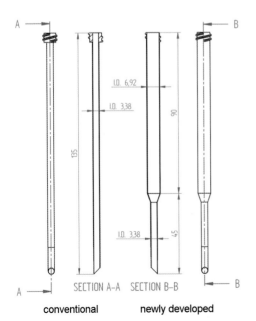

Fig. 7. Geometry of a conventional 8-gauge cannula (**A**) compared with the newly developed cannula (**B**)

contributes to a decrease in the injection pressure. Thus, more viscous cements can be injected and the risk of insufficient filling of the vertebral body is reduced. There is a need for further studies before the new cannula can be used in clinical operations.

Acknowledgments

This work was supported by the Canadian Institute of Health Research (grant no. MOP 57835), the Natural Science and Engineering Research Council and the Fonds Québecois de recherche sur la nature et les technologies (FQRNT). Images in Fig. 2 were provided by D. Chandelier, a PhD student at the biomechanics laboratory.

Glossary

Term	Explanation
Injection pressure	Total pressure needed to inject the cement into a vertebra
Injection volume	Volume of cement that is injected into the vertebra
Extravertebral pressure	Pressure necessary to overcome friction between the cement and the cannula wall
Intravertebral pressure	Pressure required for dispersion of cement in the cavities of the spongiosa and for displacement of bone marrow
Infiltration pressure	Pressure required to infiltrate the trabecular cavities
Viscosity	Toughness of fluids – in this case, cement
Extravasation	Cement leakage out of a vertebra
8-gauge	Measuring unit for the inner diameter of the cannula (corresponds to 3.38 mm)
Palm Pilot	Recorder for electronically measured data

References

Baroud G, Steffen T (2005) A new cannula to ease cement injection during vertebroplasty. Eur Spine J 14(5): 474–9

Baroud G, Bohner M, Heini P, et al (2004a) Injection biomechanics of bone cements used in vertebroplasty. Biomed Mater Eng 14: 487–504

Baroud G, Falk R, Crookshank M, et al (2004b) Experimental and theoretical investigation of the directional permeability of cancellous bone for cement infiltration. J Biomech 37(2): 189–96

Baroud G, Martin PL, Cabana F (2006) Ex-vivo experiments of a new injection instrument for vertebroplasty. Spine 31(1): 115–9

Baroud G, Vant C, Giannitsios D, et al (2005) Effect of vertebral shell on injection pressure and intravertebral pressure in vertebroplasty. Spine 30(1): 68–74

Baroud G, Wu J, Bohner M, et al (2003) How to determine the permeability for cement infiltration into osteoporotic cancellous bone. Med Eng Phys 25(4): 283–8

Bohner M, Gasser B, Baroud G, et al (2003) Theoretical and experimental model to describe the injection of a polymethylmethacrylate cement into a porous structure. Biomaterials 24: 2731–8

Cotten A, Dewatre F, Cortet B, et al (1996) Percutaneous vertebroplasty for osteolytic metastases and myeloma: effect of the percentage of lesion filling and the leakage of methyl methacrylate at clinical follow-up. Radiology 200: 525–30

Deramond H, Depriester C, Galibert P, et al (1998) Percutaneous vertebroplasty with polymethylmethacrylate. Radiol Clin North Am 36(3): 533–46

Heini PF, Berlemann U, Kaufmann M, et al (2001) Augmentation of mechanical properties in osteoporotic vertebral bones – a biomechanical investigation of vertebroplasty efficacy with different bone cements. Eur Spine J 10(2): 164–71

Heini PF, Walchli B, Berlemann U (2000) Percutaneous transpedicular vertebroplasty with PMMA: operative technique and early results. A prospective study for the treatment of osteoporotic compression fractures. Eur Spine J 9(5): 445–50

Jensen ME, Evans AJ, Mathis JM, et al (1997) Percutaneous polymethylmethacrylate vertebroplasty in the treatment of osteoporotic vertebral body compression fractures: technical aspects. Am J Neuroradiol 18(10): 1897–904

Krause WR, Miller J, Ng P (1982) The viscosity of acrylic bone cements. J Biomed Mater Res 16(3): 219–43

Mathis JM, Barr JD, Belkoff SM, et al (2001) Percutaneous vertebroplasty: a developing standard of care for vertebral compression fractures. Am J Neuroradiol 22(2): 373–81

Naumann EA, Fong KE, Keaveny TM (1999) Dependence of intertrabecular permeability on flow direction and anatomic site. Ann Biomed Eng 27(4): 517–24

San Millan Ruiz D, Burkhardt K, Jean B, et al (1999) Pathology findings with acrylic implants. Bone 25(2): 85S–90S

Wilson DR, Myers ER, Mathis JM, et al (2000) Effect of augmentation on the mechanics of the vertebral wedge fractures. Spine 25(2): 158–65

Biomechanics of vertebral cement augmentation: risk of adjacent fractures following vertebroplasty

G. Baroud and S. Wolf

Summary

Vertebroplasty is a minimally invasive procedure designed to treat osteoporotic compression fractures of vertebral bodies. In this procedure, the affected vertebral bodies are strengthened with bone cement.

New clinical and biomechanical tests have shown the appearance of new fractures in abutting vertebrae following vertebroplasty. Several hypotheses have been suggested concerning the cause of this phenomenon. In this article, we concentrate on the biomechanical hypothesis, which is based on the stiffening of osteoporotic bone as a result of cement augmentation.

It seems that under certain circumstances vertebroplasty works against itself, because it destabilizes the abutting vertebrae and causes new fractures. Although this hypothesis on the origin of compression fractures is substantiated by an increasing amount of proof, caution is still required. Vertebroplasty is a relatively new procedure, and more investigations are needed to establish the true cause of adjacent fractures.

Introduction

At the present time, more and more people are simultaneously reaching older ages, with the result that diseases such as osteoporosis are more prevalent and require greater attention. The most frequent complications of osteoporosis are compression fractures of vertebral bodies, which represent 45% of osteoporotic fractures. These fractures are often noncritical but they can result in acute pain and a decrease in the solidity and stability of the backbone.

Vertebroplasty aims to stabilize the fractured vertebral body and, if possible, completely restore its solidity, thereby alleviating pain. To achieve this aim, bone cement is injected into the vertebral body, under fluoroscopy, thereby in situ increasing both the solidity and stiffness of the vertebral body [Heini et al. 2001; Belkoff et al. 2000; Belkoff et al. 2001; Belkoff et al. 2002; Dean et al. 2000]. Vertebroplasty is not only an inexpensive alternative to conventional methods of treatment but also demonstrates many encouraging clinical successes when its increasing role in patient care is considered [Watts et al. 2001].

The present guidelines for vertebroplasty concentrate on the principle of maximizing the solidity and stiffness of the fractured vertebra by injecting the maximum volume of bone cement. However, biomechanical experiments have shown that this principle requires re-evaluation under certain circumstances, because the possible risk for an adjacent fracture has not been taken into consideration [Berlemann 2002].

Adjacent fractures are new compression fractures that occur in vertebrae adjacent to augmented vertebral bodies shortly after a vertebroplasty procedure. This phenomenon has been demonstrated in several clinical studies.

Nevertheless, despite the risk of new vertebral compression fractures, one should not lose sight of the main effect of vertebroplasty, which is to improve the stability of the fractured vertebral body [Watts et al. 2001; Heini et al. 2001; Belkoff et al. 2000, 2001, 2002; Dean et al. 2000] thus protecting it from a continuous loss of height.

Methods and results

To conduct a study on the stabilizing effect of vertebroplasty, three models with different degrees of isolation were chosen: (a) an intravertebral model, (b) a model of one vertebral body, and (c) a multisegment model.

The intravertebral model consists of one cancellous bone core with standardized dimensions and provides an opportunity to look at interactions between bones and cement without their being influenced by other anatomical factors such as the presence of the vertebral shell. The more complex model of one vertebral body is used for evaluation of the biomechanical efficiency of the procedure in relation to regeneration of fractured vertebrae and prevention of further fractures. The purpose of the multisegment model is to analyze the effect of vertebroplasty on bordering structures. These models consist of two neighboring vertebrae and the intermediate spinal disk – a functional back bone unit.

The efficiency of cement filling in terms of increasing the solidity of osteoporotic bone has been proven in the intravertebral model [Baroud et al. 2001; Baroud et al. 2003] and the model of one vertebral body [Heini et al. 2001; Belkoff et al. 2000, 2001, 2002; Dean et al. 2000]. In contrast, results based on the multisegmental model challenge the principle of maximized filling, because this can be disadvantageous for neighboring vertebrae [Berlemann et al. 2002].

The vertebral shell is essential for the solidity and stability of a healthy vertebral body, and a fracture through the shell results in partial loss of this stabilizing factor [Rockoff et al. 1969]. Although the augmentation aspires to restore the solidity of the vertebral body, only the trabecular rack and not the vertebral shell is stabilized. The result is a kind of intravertebral pillar made of cement.

Experimental single vertebra models, mainly osteoporotic, generally test the biomechanical stability of cadaveric vertebrae in axial compression (Fig. 8) prior to and following vertebroplasty. Excised cadaveric vertebrae are augmented with bone cement, following the maximal filling paradigm, and samples then undergo biomechanical testing using a universal materials testing machine [Heini et al. 2001].

Results of biomechanical tests show that a healthy vertebral body can withstand 10 times more axial compression than a strong osteoporotic vertebral body [Heini et al. 2001] (Fig. 9). Vertebroplasty tries to rebuild this strength.

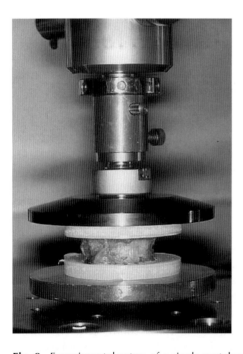

Fig. 8. Experimental setup of a single vertebral model [Heini et al. 2001] in axial compression on a universal testing machine. Most biomechanical testing is performed in axial compression because it is the direction of the greatest loading on the spine

The ability of cement augmentation to stabilize osteoporotic bone in the vertebral body seems indisputable; it is possible to rebuild the solidity to the same level as that of intact bone, and even more. However, the following questions arise from these studies: What is effective repair? How much strength and stiffness should be restored to the vertebral body?

The ideal level of restoration is unknown; strength can be restored to a prefracture intact level or to a healthy nonosteoporotic level. Until the ideal level is determined, augmentations may be excessive, and reports suggest that these may have adverse biomechanical effects on the surrounding tissues. Specifically, studies suggest that vertebroplasty may cause adjacent fractures (Fig. 10).

Recent clinical studies have supported these observations, demonstrating significantly increased risk for adjacent fractures. Uppin et al. [Uppin et al. 2003] reported that two-thirds of observed new fractures occurred within 30 days after a vertebroplasty procedure. Similarly, Grados et al. [Grados et al. 2000] reported an increased odds ratio for the appearance of adjacent vertebral fractures prior to (1.44) and post (2.27) augmentation. Legroux-Gérot et al. [2004] noted a similar increase in the odds ratio. More recently, Kim et al. [2004] reported that 8% of all vertebrae in their study developed new fractures following vertebroplasty, thus also suggesting that vertebroplasty increases the risk of adjacent fractures.

From these findings, it is important not only to notice the significance of these studies but also to understand the underlying mechanisms. If a mechanism can be found to explain the appearance of adjacent vertebral fractures, it may be possible to alter the treatment to prevent this possibly harmful long-term effect.

Several hypotheses for the appearance of adjacent vertebral fractures have been suggested. A *first hypothesis* by Ross et al. [1993], and others more recently [Heini and Orler 2004; Lindsay et al. 2001; Fribourg et al. 2004], suggests that it is the effect of the natural progression of osteoporosis. This is reasonable, because the risk of subsequent fractures increases by four times following the appearance of an initial vertebral fracture, even without vertebroplasty.

A *second hypothesis* by Uppin et al. [2003] and Heini et al. [2004] suggests that new fractures result from the increased level of activity of patients following a vertebroplasty procedure. It is postulated

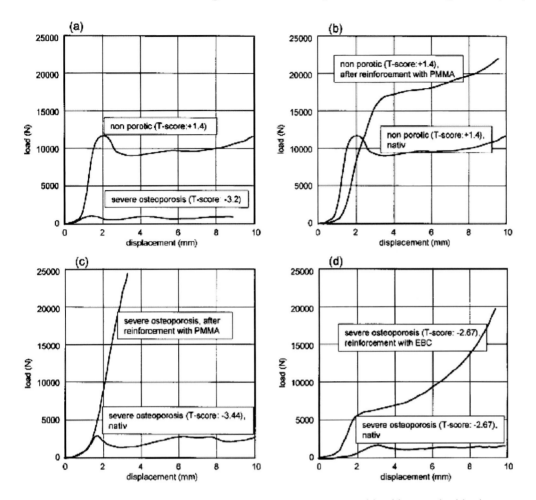

Fig. 9. Qualitative load-displacement curves representing untreated healthy vertebral bodies; untreated osteoporotic vertebral bodies; and augmented osteoporotic vertebral bodies, with maximal filling with experimental brushite cement [Heini et al. 2001]

that the increased physical activity places increased stress on the vertebrae, causing them to fracture. Again, this is feasible, because patients generally experience remarkable pain relief following a vertebroplasty procedure.

Although these two hypotheses are both reasonable, neither allows for any hope of improving the situation and minimizing this undesirable effect.

A *third hypothesis* was proposed by Baroud et al. [2001, 2003]; namely, that perhaps vertebroplasty itself is the cause of these fractures, as a result of its biomechanical effects on the surrounding tissues. This is a two-part hypothesis, which proposes that

(a) the rigid cement filling of vertebroplasty leads to increased stiffness of the augmented vertebra; and

(b) this, in turn, produces increased loading in the adjacent vertebrae.

Examination of the third hypothesis by both experimental and computational means is the focus of this chapter. Specifically, experimental tests examined part (a) through materials tests, and computational analyses examined part (b) using multisegment models.

Baroud et al. [2001] conducted experimental materials testing on cylindrical samples (height and diameter ~8.4 ± 1.6 mm) comprising three experimental groups: acrylic bone cement, calcium phosphate bone cement, and osteoporotic bone samples – both untreated and augmented using acrylic bone cement. The cylindrical samples were subjected to axial compression between parallel plates, and the

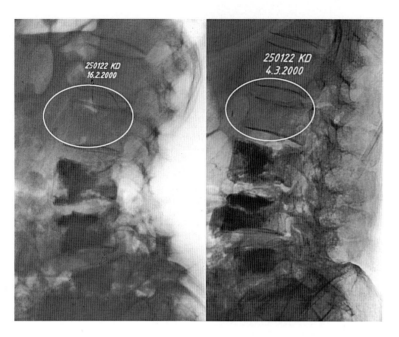

Fig. 10. A typical case of an adjacent vertebral fracture. The radiograph on the left was taken prior to the vertebroplasty procedure, and the radiograph on the right was taken 2 weeks after the procedure. Comparison of the two radiographs demonstrates the appearance of an adjacent vertebral fracture (highlighted). The radiographs are from the same patient [Baroud et al. 2003]

elastic modulus and ultimate strength were measured.

The specific findings on the elastic modulus of the intravertebral model (Fig. 11) were reported. There were only minor differences in the elastic properties within each group of cement and between these two cement types. However, it was evident that large differences exist between the cement and the bone; cement is much stiffer than bone. Finally, the most important finding was that augmented osteoporotic bone is *12 times stiffer* than untreated osteoporotic bone.

Similarly, the main findings were reported in relation to the ultimate strength of the osteoporotic bone (Fig. 12). Only minor differences exist between each type of cement; however, larger differences exist between the two groups. More importantly, an even greater difference exists between the untreated osteoporotic bone and the augmented osteoporotic bone: following augmentation, the osteoporotic bone is *36 times stronger*, an important increase in its load-bearing capacity.

These results demonstrated a substantial change in the material properties of trabecular bone following augmentation and support the hypothesis by confirming (a): augmentation leads to an increased stiffness in the augmented cancellous bone. From this, it is hypothesized that increased stiffness will lead to reduction in intravertebral joint flexibility and increase in disc pressure.

Experimental biomechanical studies are limited in their use and therefore computational studies are often conducted to complement them. Computa-

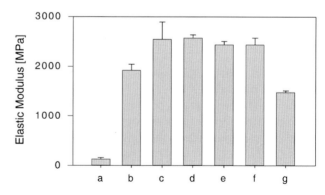

Fig. 11. The modulus of elasticity of three groups of cylindrical samples: (**a**) untreated osteoporotic cancellous bone, (**b**) Biopex cement, (**c**) Norian SRS cement, (**d**) vertebroplastic cement, (**e**) cranioplastic cement, (**f**) Simplex cement, and (**g**) osteoporotic cancellous bone infiltrated with cement

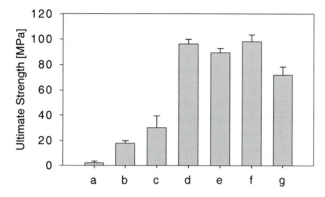

Fig. 12. The ultimate strength of three groups of cylindrical samples: (**a**) untreated osteoporotic cancellous bone, (**b**) Biopex cement, (**c**) Norian SRS cement, (**d**) vertebroplastic cement (acrylic), (**e**) cranioplastic cement (acrylic), (**f**) Simplex cement (acrylic), and (**g**) osteoporotic cancellous bone infiltrated with cement

tional studies employ a technique called finite element (FE) modeling, a tool used by engineers to examine stress and strain fields in complex structures; these are especially valuable because they have the power to show hidden effects, such as the mechanisms responsible for observed phenomena.

Baroud et al. [2003] and Polikeit et al. [2003] created a computational model to examine the loading in both augmented and non-augmented motion segments. The basic FE model was of a functional spinal unit (FSU) composed of two lumbar vertebrae and one intervertebral disc. Each component was composed of several parts: the vertebrae consisted of an internal cancellous bone structure enclosed by a cortical shell, and the disc was a water-like nucleus surrounded by fibrous rings and a Teflon-like annulus. The augmented FSU was altered to model the reinforcement of the lower, L5, vertebra with bone cement.

Each material was modeled separately to ensure a more accurate representation of the *in vivo* environment. The bone was modeled as a linearly elastic material. The nucleus was an incompressible solid with nonlinear material properties, the surrounding fibers were nonlinear rings, and the annulus was linearly elastic. Both the augmented and nonaugmented FSU models were distally constrained and subjected to axial compression.

The resulting mechanical loading (Fig. 13) was then examined for each case to determine how the augmentation altered loading in the surrounding tis-

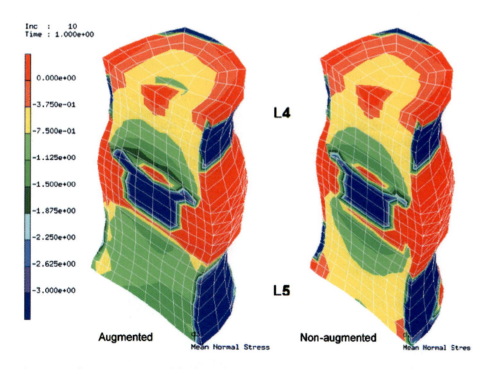

Fig. 13. Multisegment FE model where the mean stresses (MPa) in the sagittal plane highlight the load shift. The endplates of the untreated model (right) bulge symmetrically under nucleus pressure. The rigid cement pillar in L5 inhibits the inward endplate bulge of the superior L5 endplate in the augmented model (left). This increases both the inward endplate bulge of the inferior L4 endplate and the bone stresses in L4 [Baroud et al. 2003]

sues. The broad finding was that there is a redistribution of pressure in the augmented model.

Closer examination of the pressures shows several important changes. There was a significant increase in intravertebral disc pressure (19%), an increased load on L4 (17%), and an increase in joint flexibility (11%). In addition, there was a decrease in the endplate bulge of the superior endplate of L5 and a resulting increase in the endplate bulge of the inferior endplate of L4. These findings represent an important change in the mechanical loading of the augmented model [Berlemann et al. 2002].

Biomechanical cadaveric studies in spinal motion segments have shown that both the intravertebral disc and the endplates determine flexibility. For a nonaugmented joint, it has been reported that the intravertebral disc contributes approximately two-thirds of the flexibility, and the endplates contribute approximately one-third, or about 15% per endplate [Brinckmann et al. 1983].

Vertebroplasty seems to alter normal joint loading through reinforcement of the vertebral body with rigid cement in a mechanism termed the pillar effect. The augmentation creates a pillar of cement that reduces flexibility of the endplate by inhibiting endplate bulge, thereby reducing flexibility of the entire motion segment. This decreased flexibility may cause loading to be redistributed, thereby increasing loading on adjacent vertebrae.

These computational results thereby confirm part (b) of the biomechanical hypothesis; that is, the rigid pillar effect of the cement creates increased loading in adjacent vertebrae.

Results obtained in the multisegment model suggest a *mechanism* responsible for the change in biomechanical loading leading to adjacent vertebral fractures: the pillar effect, outlined in the following steps:

1. Augmentation with rigid cement produces *increased stiffness* in the augmented vertebra.
2. Increased stiffness in the augmented vertebra *reduces its endplate bulge*.
3. Reduction in endplate bulge is responsible for *reducing overall joint flexibility*.
4. The reduction in joint flexibility seeks to reverse itself by *increasing the intervertebral disc pressure*.
5. The increased *intervertebral* disc pressure seeks to relieve itself by *increasing the load on the adjacent vertebra*.
6. The increased load on the adjacent vertebra relates directly to *increased risk of fracture*.

Discussion

Further evidence to suggest the pillar effect as the mechanism responsible for adjacent vertebral fractures has been reported in the literature in support of the findings previously presented.

Ananthakrishnan et al. [2003] were the first to experimentally measure disc pressure, an important step that provides the first evidence of increased loading in surrounding tissues. These authors concluded that the significantly increased intervertebral disc pressure following augmentation is communicated via the disc to the adjacent vertebra.

Berlemann et al. [2002] conducted experimental studies on FSUs and reported a 19% decrease in overall strength of the FSU following vertebroplasty when compared with matched controls. Further, these authors reported that failure was isolated to the untreated cranial vertebra in the augmented FSUs, whereas failure generally occurred in both vertebrae in the untreated control FSUs.

In experimental studies on multisegment models, Lu et al. [2001] found that stiffness increased above the level of intact models, but that after cyclic loading stiffness is brought back below the level of intact FSUs.

Wilcox [2004], using FE modeling of a fractured model, concluded that a load shift to the untreated vertebra in an FSU pair was responsible for instigating new compression fractures. The fractured model was subjected to a 16% increase in strain in the adjacent vertebra. The presence of increased loading in this vertebra turned it into the weakest link in the model, thus creating a venue for the continued increase in loading until failure occurred in the form of a new compression fracture. Polikeit et al. [2003], using an elaborate multisegment FE model, reported similar results.

The three most important findings drawn from research on adjacent vertebral fractures are as follows:

1. Although rigid cement augmentation increases the strength of an individual vertebra, it seems to weaken the spine as a whole;
2. vertebroplasty seems to result in increased loading in tissues adjacent to the augmented vertebra; and
3. the mechanism responsible for the load increase in the surrounding tissues, especially the adjacent vertebrae, is the pillar effect.

Thus, it appears that the pillar effect contributes to the risk of adjacent vertebral fractures, and therefore the next logical step is to apply this knowledge to improving vertebroplasty by preventing the appearance of new fractures following the procedure.

Currently, the mechanical properties of bone and cement are drastically different. It has been suggested that cements could be adapted to more closely resemble the properties of bone as a possible solution to the risk of adjacent vertebral fractures. Young's modulus and the ultimate strength can be decreased from normal cement values to match those of bone.

Using computational models, Wilcox [2004] and Sun and Liebschner [2004] have both demonstrated that the excess loading on adjacent vertebrae can be altered through the use of less-stiff materials. The cement's porosity can be increased by altering its composition through the addition of soluble fillers or other materials not currently in use. An example of a successful adjustment is provided by De Wijn et al. [1976], who were able to decrease the compressive strength of cement from 80 MPa to approximately 5 MPa through the addition of a 65 vol% aqueous phase.

A further method for improving the mechanical loading response is to change the current paradigm from maximal filling to minimal filling. Berlemann et al. [2002] have reported a negative correlation between cement volume and the overall strength of an experimental FSU, an indication of the importance of minimal filling. More specifically, Belkoff et al. [2001] reported that their experimental models were adequately augmented after injecting only 2 cc of bone cement, and Liebschner et al. [2001] reported that injecting only 3.5 cc of cement adequately stabilized their computational models.

To successfully implement the use of either modified cements or an adapted minimal-filling paradigm in vertebroplasty, further studies, particularly clinical studies, are required. Specifically, the minimum strength and stiffness required to afford sufficient stability to fractured vertebrae, while also providing an appropriate mechanical response in the surrounding tissues of the spine, must be determined.

Although there is an increasing amount of evidence to support this theory of the origin of adjacent fractures, caution is needed. Vertebroplasty is a relatively new procedure and further observations are required to conclusively determine the cause of adjacent fractures.

References

Ananthakrishnan D, Lotz JC, Berven S, Puttlitz C (2003) Changes in spinal loading due to vertebral augmentation: vertebroplasty versus kyphoplasty. Annual Meeting of the American Academy of Orthopaedic Surgeons, New Orleans, p 472

Baroud G, Goerke U, Beckman L, Steffen T (2001) Physical changes of the vertebral tissue treated with vertebroplasty. XVIIIth Congress of International Society of Biomechanics, Zurich, p 728

Baroud G, Nemes J, Ferguson S, Steffen T (2003) Material changes in osteoporotic human cancellous bone following infiltration with acrylic bone cement for a vertebral cement augmentation. Comput Meth in Biomechan Biomed Eng 6(2): 133–9

Baroud G, Nemes J, Heini P, Steffen T (2003) Load shift of the intervertebral disc after a vertebroplasty: a finite-element study. Eur Spine J 12(4): 421–6

Belkoff SM, Mathis JM, Erbe EM, Fenton DC (2000) Biomechanical evaluation of a new bone cement for use in vertebroplasty. Spine 25(9): 1061–4

Belkoff SM, Mathis JM, Jasper LE, Deramond H (2001) The biomechanics of vertebroplasty. The effect of cement volume on mechanical behaviour. Spine 26(14): 1537–41

Belkoff SM, Mathis JM, Jasper LE (2002) Ex vivo biomechanical comparison of hydroxyapatite and polymethylmethacrylate cements for use with vertebroplasty. AJNR Am J Neuroradiol 23(10): 1647–51

Berlemann U, Ferguson SJ, Nolte LP, Heini PF (2002) Adjacent vertebral failure after vertebroplasty. A biomechanical investigation. J Bone Joint Surg Br 84(5): 748–52

Brinckmann P, Frobin W, Hierholzer E, Horst M (1983) Deformation of the vertebral end-plate under axial loading of the spine. Spine 8(8): 851–6

De Wijn JR (1976) Poly(methyl methacrylate)-aqueous phase blends: in situ curing porous materials. J Biomed Mater Res 10(4): 625–35

Dean JR, Ison KT, Gishen P (2000) The strengthening effect of percutaneous vertebroplasty. Clin Radiol 55(6): 471–6

Fribourg D, Tang C, Sra P, Delamarter R, Bae H (2004) Incidence of subsequent vertebral fracture after kyphoplasty. Spine 29(20): 2270–76

Grados F, Depriester C, Cayrolle G, Hardy N, Deramond H, Fardellone P (2000) Long-term observations of vertebral osteoporotic fractures treated by percutaneous vertebroplasty. Rheumatology (Oxford) 39(12): 1410–4

Heini PF, Berlemann U, Kaufmann M, Lippuner K, Fankhauser C, van Landuyt P (2001) Augmentation of mechanical properties in osteoporotic vertebral bones – a biomechanical investigation of vertebroplasty efficacy with different bone cement. Eur Spine J 10(2): 164–71

Heini PF, Orler R (2004) Vertebroplastik bei hochgradiger Osteoporose. Technik und Erfahrung mit plurisegmentalen Injektionen. Orthopäde 33(1): 22–30

Kim SH, Kang HS, Choi J-A, Ahn JM (2004) Risk factors of new compression fractures in adjacent vertebrae after percutaneous vertebroplasty. Acta Radiologica 45(4): 440–5(6)

Legroux-Gerot I, Lormeau C, Boutry N, Cotten A, Duquesnoy B, Cortet B (2004) Long-term follow-up of vertebral osteoporotic fractures treated by percutaneous vertebroplasty. Clin Rheumatol 23(4): 310–7

Liebschner MA, Rosenberg WS, Keaveny TM (2001) Effects of bone cement volume and distribution on vertebral stiffness after vertebroplasty. Spine 26(14): 1547–54

Lindsay R, Silverman SL, Cooper C, Hanley DA, Barton I, Broy SB, Licata A, Benhamou L, Geusens P, et al (2001) Risk of new vertebral fracture in the year following a fracture. Jama 285(3): 320–3

Lu WW, Cheung KM, Li YW, Luk KD, Holmes AD, Zhu QA, Leong JC (2001) Bioactive bone cement as a principal fixture for spinal burst fracture: an in vitro biomechanical and morphologic study. Spine 26(2): 2684–90; discussion 2690–1

Polikeit A, Nolte LP, Ferguson SJ (2003) The effect of cement augmentation on the load transfer in an osteoporotic functional spinal unit: finite-element analysis. Spine 28(10): 991–6

Rockoff SD, Sweet E, Bleustein J (1969) The relative contribution of trabecular and cortical bone strength to the strength of human lumbar vertebrae. Calcif Tissue Res 3: 163–75

Rohlmann A, Zander T, Jony A, Weber U, Bergmann G (2005) Einfluss der Wirbelkörpersteifigkeit vor und nach der Vertebroplastik auf den intradiskalen Druck. Biomed Technik 50(5): 148–52

Ross PD, Genant HK, Davis JW, Miller PD, Wasnich RD (1993) Predicting vertebral fracture incidence from prevalent fractures and bone density among non-black, osteoporotic women. Osteoporos Int 3(3): 120–6

Sun K, Liebschner AK (2004) Evolution of vertebroplasty: a biomechanical perspective. Annals of Biomed Eng 32(1): 77–91

Uppin AA, Hirsch JA, Centenera LV, Pfiefer BA, Pazianos AG, Choi IS (2003) Occurrence of new vertebral body fracture after percutaneous vertebroplasty in patients with osteoporosis. Radiology 226(1): 119–24

Watts NB, Harris, ST, Genant HK (2001) Treatment of painful osteoporotic vertebral fractures with percutaneous vertebroplasty or kyphoplasty. Osteoporos Int 12(6): 429–37

Wilcox RK (2004) Do vertebroplasty cements have the optimum mechanical properties? Transactions of 7th World Biomaterials Congress, Sydney, Abstract 1547

Chapter 5

Indications, contraindications and imaging in balloon kyphoplasty

S. Becker

Indications and contraindications

Balloon kyphoplasty has now been carried out worldwide on over 230,000 patients with more than 275,000 vertebral fractures. As with every technique, the best results are achieved if the special indications and contraindications are strictly adhered to.

The technique of balloon kyphoplasty was initially developed in 1998 for osteoporotic compression fractures of vertebral bodies, but with the spread of the technique the indication has now been extended to tumors and traumatic fractures.

The indications with the best experience are painful osteoporotic compression fractures of the thoracic and lumbar spine resulting from primary or secondary osteoporosis. Further indications concern tumor metastasis, to which we have devoted a special chapter (see Chapter 9).

Increasing experience has allowed the use of balloon kyphoplasty on traumatic or osteoporotic compression fractures of vertebral bodies of the chest and the lumbar spine; however, we recommend starting with kyphotic and osteoporotic spinal fractures.

As experience in trauma treatment has increased, there are hardly any strict contraindications against the operation, apart from general contraindications such as coagulation disorder, unsuitability for general or local anesthesia, or the inability to lie in a prone position. Before performing a balloon kyphoplasty it is necessary to clarify whether the fracture is primarily osteoporotic or is a traumatic fracture of an osteoporotic bone. It must also be clarified in advance whether the pain that the patient experiences is caused by the fracture (see Chapter 9).

Severe iodine allergy is a special contraindication; the balloons are normally filled with iodine-based contrast medium and in principle can burst, therefore undiluted gadolinium should be used in the presence of a severe iodine allergy. Nevertheless, if a balloon does burst it will remain whole and there is merely a small perforation from which the contents (contrast medium) are emptied, i.e. the balloon does not fragment.

As already remarked, the contraindications have changed as the result of increasing experience and broader indication. Only a few years ago, balloon kyphoplasty on people under the age of 40 was contraindicated, but this no longer applies. The development of new bone cements means that balloon kyphoplasty can perfectly well be performed on those under 40; however, we use absorbable bone substitution materials with these patients (see respective chapters on resorbable bone cements).

Imaging

Imaging plays a crucial role in the diagnosis of osteoporosis, apart from the clinical symptoms listed in Chapter 3.

The locally experienced pain means that a suspected fracture can often be pin-pointed in clinical examination. However, an x-ray with anterior-posterior and lateral views does not always show the fracture and is even less likely to permit determination of its age. Furthermore, it is possible that renewed sintering in the same segment of an already existing fracture has taken place. The diagnosis is made much more difficult if no earlier x-rays are available.

MRI thus plays the decisive role in the diagnosis of osteoporotic fractures and the differentiation from metastatic fractures [Baker 1990; Baur 1998; Chan 2002; Park 2004; Stabler 1992]. When making the diagnosis from MRI, it is important to take the case history of the patient into account. If the patient is suspected of already having an old fracture, it could well be that the normal T1 and T2 sequences cannot show the acute fracture on the MRI.

In general, the T1 sequence shows a reduced signal in the case of an acute fracture; in contrast, the T2 sequence shows an increased signal because of the fracture edema. After a few months this can differ individually; the T2 examination increasingly loses its edema characteristic, so that an extended fat suppression will be needed. Fat suppression of the T2 image, known as short tau inverted recovery (STIR), is particularly indicated in the presence of occult fractures, unclear x-ray results or older fractures [Meyers 1991; Van Gelderen 1997]. There will always be a positive STIR sequence in cases of osteoporotic fracture [Gaitanis 2004]. As is shown in the example (Fig. 14), a fracture edema can be traced up to a year or more. In case of older osteoporotic changes we always recommend MRI using the STIR sequence, because only this can ensure that the height of the fracture is diagnosed correctly and that the operation will be limited to the appropriate segment.

MRI examinations have considerably gained in importance; formerly, whenever a fissure was suspected or if a fracture could not be clearly identified on an x-ray, conservative treatment was started and, in order to diagnose the further course with increasing collapse, the fracture was x-rayed again 4 to 6 weeks later. Thus, connection with an accident or a suspected fissure could be verified retrospectively. This method is no longer usual practice; it is now recommended that the MRI is done at an early stage. Indeed, it is inadvisable to perform a balloon kyphoplasty without an MRI, otherwise there is a risk of kyphoplasting the wrong segment.

If it is not possible to get an MRI, because of contraindications (e.g. existing pacemaker), a combination of computer tomography and bone scan would be the alternative [Cook 2002; Ryan 1997; Wiener 1998]. If there is a traumatic genesis (a traumatic fracture in a patient with osteoporosis), it is recommended that the guidelines of trauma surgery are followed and additional computer tomography performed when a posterior wall fracture is suspected.

For diagnosing fractures of the spine, computer tomography has a lower sensitivity than MRI [Rhee 2002] and can confirm the diagnosis only in combination with bone scintigraphy. The latter, however, has a diagnostic window: the scintigraphy can be falsely negative in the acute phase following the fracture, and an already healed fracture can still show as positive years after the event. The sensitivity here is also considerably lower than on MRI [Ryan 1994; Wiener 1998]. PET examination can also confirm the diagnosis in case of doubt [Schmitz 2002].

In summary, before performing balloon kyphoplasty an x-ray in two planes and an MRI (if possible with a STIR sequence) should be routinely carried out. This approach significantly increases the sensitivity and specificity of the methods. In our daily practice we perform balloon kyphoplasty only if the clinical symptoms and the localization of the height coincide with the findings of the MRI and X-ray.

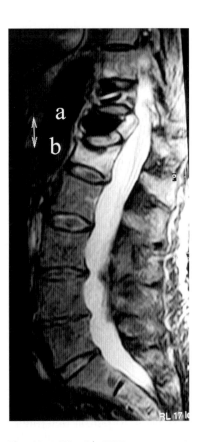

Fig. 14. MRI with STIR sequence 4 months after treatment of fractures of T11 and T12 with balloon kyphoplasty (**a**) refracture 4 weeks after initial treatment. The MRI clearly shows both the 4 months old fracture as well as the acuter, 4 weeks old fracture (**b**)

References

Baker LL, Goodman SB, Perkash I, Lane B, Enzmann DR (1990) Benign versus pathologic compression fractures of vertebral bodies: assessment with conventional spin-echo, chemical-shift, and STIR MR imaging. Radiology 174(2): 495–502

Baur A, Stabler A, Bruning R, Bartl R, Krodel A, Reiser M, Deimling M (1998) Diffusion-weighted MR imaging of bone marrow: differentiation of benign versus pathologic compression fractures. Radiology 207(2): 349–56

Chan JH, Peh WC, Tsui EY, Chau LF, Cheung KK, Chan KB, Yuen MK, Wong ET, Wong KP (2002) Acute vertebral body compression fractures: discrimination between benign and malignant causes using apparent diffusion coefficients. Br J Radiol 75(891): 207–14

Cook GJ, Hannaford E, See M, Clarke SE, Fogelman I (2002) The value of bone scintigraphy in the evaluation of osteoporotic patients with back pain. Scand J Rheumatol 31(4): 245–8

Gaitanis IN, Hadjipavlou AG, Katonis PG, Tzermiadianos MN, Pasku DS, Patwardhan AG (2004) Balloon kyphoplasty for the treatment of pathological vertebral compressive fractures. Eur Spine J 8

Meyers SP, Wiener SN (1991) Magnetic resonance imaging features of fractures using the short tau inversion recovery (STIR) sequence: correlation with radiographic findings. Skeletal Radiol 20(7): 499–507

Park SW, Lee JH, Ehara S, Park YB, Sung SO, Choi JA, Joo YE (2004) Single shot fast spin echo diffusion-weighted MR imaging of the spine; Is it useful in differentiating malignant metastatic tumor infiltration from benign fracture edema? Clin Imaging 28(2): 102–8

Rhee PM, Bridgeman A, Acosta JA, Kennedy S, Wang DS, Sarveswaran J, Rhea JT (2002) Lumbar fractures in adult blunt trauma: axial and single-slice helical abdominal and pelvic computed tomographic scans versus portable plain films. J Trauma 53(4): 663–7

Ryan PJ, Fogelman I (1997) Bone scintigraphy in metabolic bone disease. Semin Nucl Med 27(3): 291–305

Ryan PJ, Fogelman I (1994) Osteoporotic vertebral fractures: diagnosis with radiography and bone scintigraphy. Radiology 190(3): 669–72

Schmitz A, Risse JH, Textor J, Zander D, Biersack HJ, Schmitt O, Palmedo H (2002) FDG-PET findings of vertebral compression fractures in osteoporosis: preliminary results. Osteoporos Int 13(9): 755–61

Stabler A, Krimmel K, Seiderer M, Gartner C, Fritsch S, Raum W (1992) The nuclear magnetic resonance tomographic differentiation of osteoporotic and tumor-related vertebral fractures. The value of subtractive TR gradient-echo sequences, STIR sequences and Gd-DTPA. Rofo 157(3): 215–21

Van Gelderen WF, al-Hindawi M, Gale RS, Steward AH, Archibald CG (1997) Significance of short tau inversion recovery magnetic resonance sequence in the management of skeletal injuries. Australas Radiol 41 (1): 13–5

Wiener SN, Neumann DR, Rzeszotarski MS (1989) Comparison of magnetic resonance imaging and radionuclide bone imaging of vertebral fractures. Clin Nucl Med 14(9): 666–70

Sequential therapy after osteoporotic vertebral fracture – a treatment scheme

As shown above, vertebroplasty and balloon kyphoplasty have been extensively investigated in various health technology assessments (HTA) in different countries. Benefits, pros and cons have been discussed, but is there still a place for conservative treatment of osteoporotic vertebral fractures?

Worldwide, conservative treatment is still the gold standard even 20 years after the introduction of vertebroplasty and nearly 10 years after balloon kyphoplasty. Personal experience and multiple publications show the value of conservative treatment [Becker 2006].

However, the main complication after conservative treatment remains the risk of increased kyphosis with its detrimental impact on subsequent fractures and pulmonary function [Browner 1991; Cooper 1993; Kado 1999; Lunt 2003], as has already been shown (see Chapter 3). Therefore, after management of pain, management of kyphosis should be the center of any therapeutic focus [Becker 2006]. This goal can be realized with vertebroplasty up to six weeks after the fracture, or even longer in cases with osteonecrosis. Nevertheless, because of the time factor in vertebroplasty, some patients are treated immediately without taking into account the good results after conservative therapy, resulting sometimes in unnecessary interventions.

I have therefore adapted a concept of the Swiss Society of Spinal Surgery, whose members reached consensus on a sequential treatment plan, needed nationally for reasons of reimbursement. The plan includes conservative measures and indications of treatment failure and has been followed with success for nearly two years in our center (see Fig. 15) [Becker 2006]. The main point of interest in this scheme is the regular follow-up at the treatment center, together with an interdisciplinary approach involving the radiologist, orthopedic surgeon and medical specialist, which assures optimal treatment.

Patients should be transferred to a specialized and experienced center as soon as possible after an osteoporosis fracture, to be assessed for conservative or operative management. If the patient shows no indication for immediate balloon kyphoplasty (reduction of vertebral height > 1/3rd in relation to an adjacent healthy vertebra, kyphosis > 15° in the thoracic spine and 10° in the lumbar spine), conser-

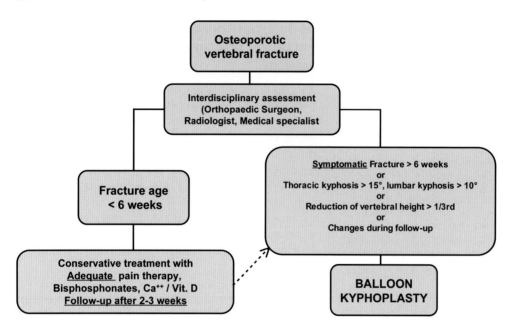

Fig. 15

vative treatment is indicated. Most centers have their own conservative treatment schemes and should therefore continue to follow the scheme that gives the best results. For lumbar or thoracolumbar fractures, we immobilize the patient in a slightly flexible lumbar brace and begin outpatient physiotherapy under adequate management of pain. If the fracture is very painful, the patient will receive treatment as an inpatient. We also assess the need for calcium, vitamin D and bisphosphonates, and as most of the patients are not under an adequate treatment scheme we start all three immediately. After two to three weeks all patients are carefully reassessed with clinical and radiological investigation in the outpatient clinic. This is the central part of the treatment scheme, as only regular follow-ups can demonstrate changes of kyphosis angles of vertebral height and failures of conservative management. Any changes of the radiological result towards the shown indication for surgery or failure of pain management or persistent pain (VAS > 3) for longer than six weeks warrant balloon kyphoplasty.

This scheme excludes immediate vertebroplasty and avoids unnecessary operations as it includes the opinion and result of conservative medicine together with balloon kyphoplasty. Because good results are achieved with balloon kyphoplasty even six weeks or more after a fracture, individual adequate treatment can be chosen according to the pain status and deformity. Immediate surgery in cases without the required parameters for balloon kyphoplasty may yield good results regarding pain, but in those cases the known risk of vertebroplasty has to be accepted, always bearing in mind that conservative management may have reached the same goal as the operation.

In orthopedic surgery nowadays it is important to develop treatment schemes that optimize and standardize the treatment and the results. A scheme is only as good as it is when transformed and adapted to individual patients, and in some cases a treatment scheme may not be applicable (e.g. patients receiving cortisone treatment or those with vertebral osteonecrosis). Nevertheless, I think that this guideline helps both the interdisciplinary team and the general practitioner to optimize the treatment of osteoporosis vertebral fracture while minimizing the risks; furthermore, the guideline recognizes the trend towards interdisciplinary approaches and discussion of budgets.

References

Becker S, Bartl R, Bretschneider W, Meissner J, Ogon M (2006) Stufentherapie bei osteoporotischer Wirbelfraktur. J Miner Stoffwechs 13(1): 27–8

Browner WS, Seeley DG, Vogt TM, Cummings S (1991) Non-trauma mortality in elderly women with low bone mineral density. Lancet 338: 355–8

Cooper C, Atkinson EJ, Jacobsen SJ, O'Fallon WM, Melton LJ 3rd (1993) Population-based study of survival after osteoporotic fractures. Am J Epidemiology 137(9): 1001–5

Kado DM, Browner WS, Palermo L, Nevitt MC, Genant HK, Cummings SR (1999) Vertebral fractures and mortality in older women. Arch Int Med 159: 1215–20

Lunt M, O'Neill TW, Felsenberg D, Reeve J, Kanis JA, Cooper C, Silman AJ (2003) European Prospective Osteoporosis Study Group. Characteristics of a prevalent vertebral deformity predict subsequent vertebral fracture: results from the European Prospective Osteoporosis Study (EPOS). Bone 33(4): 505–13

Chapter 6

Special anatomy and classification of fractures

The venous drainage system of the vertebral body and spine and its consequences for balloon kyphoplasty

S. Becker

Because of the possibility of extravasation of cement from the vertebral body, the venous system of the spine should be carefully considered. The vertebral venous system (VVS, Batson's plexus [Batson 1940]) is basically divided into three parts: the external vertebral venous system (EVVS), the basivertebral system (BS) and the internal vertebral venous system (IVVS) [Batson 1940; Clemens 1961; Fleischhauer 1994] (Fig. 16).

The vertebral venous system (Fig. 16)

In principle all vertebral venous systems are built horizontally. Each vertebral body has an outer venous plexus and also has veins running within the vertebral body. Ventrally, the outer plexus lies close to the vertebral body (plexus venosus vertebralis externus anterior), and dorsally it lies on the vertebral arches and ligaments (plexus venosus vertebralis externus posterior). This system is directly connected to the azygos vein and the thoracic hemiazygos vein, as well as to the ascending lumbar veins via the segmental lumbar veins. Thus the inferior and superior vena cavae are directly connected dorsally via this system (Fig. 17).

The basivertebral system

The basivertebral system (BS) lies within the vertebral body, and is formed either by one vein or by a pair of veins which take in smaller veins from the vertebral body. The two veins unite centrally in the basivertebral vein and connect ventrally with the anterior venous vertebral plexus and towards the spinal cord with the IVVS.

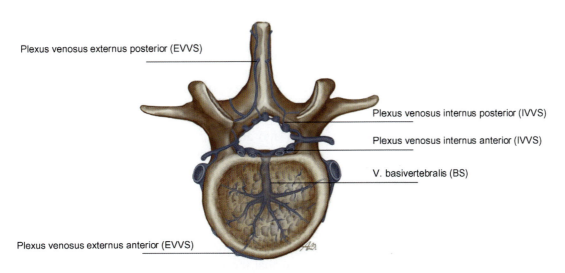

Fig. 16. The vertebral venous system and its individual parts: The external vertebral venous system (EVVS), the basivertebral system (BS) and the internal vertebral venous system (IVVS)

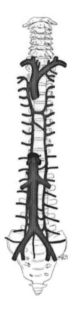

Fig. 17. Collateral circulation between inferior and the superior vena cava via the venous vertebral system

The internal vertebral venous system

The IVVS (epidural plexus) lies directly in the epidural lipoid space. In accordance with the EVVS, the IVVS also forms an anterior venous plexus (plexus venosus vertebralis internus anterior) which is directly connected to the basivertebral vein, and a posterior venous plexus (plexus venosus vertebralis internus posterior) which is directly connected to the external dorsal venous plexus. Thus there are two rings of veins (EVVS and IVVS) surrounding each vertebral body in each segment; the rings are connected via the BS.

All three systems are designed as valveless venous systems. The EVVS and IVVS run along the complete spine, from the hiatus sacralis up to the foramen magnum, and lead anteriorly into the basilar venous plexus and posteriorly into the suboccipital sinus [Groen 2004].

The volume of the venous system of the spine is 20 times larger than the arterial volume [Clemens 1961; Vogelsang 1970] and, because of the absence of valves, allows blood flow in both directions, depending on the intra-abdominal and intrathoracic pressures. The function of the inordinately large venous system of the spine is still not clear. Possible functions are: an already laid out collateral circulation in case of occlusion of a vena cava, and the possibility of compensating the venous pressure [Herlihy 1947]; a safety cushion for the medulla [Penning 1981; Reesink 2001]; an absorption space for cerebrospinal fluid [Zenker 1994]; or a cooling mechanism for the central nervous system [Zenker 1996].

The effects that the anatomy has on injection of liquid polymethylmethacrylate (PMMA) cement into the vertebral body are obvious and were shown in vivo in a study by Phillips. Contrast medium is directly instilled during balloon kyphoplasty and vertebroplasty, and it was observed that the medium leaked into the EVVS and the IVVS when using either technique, although significantly less escaped during balloon kyphoplasty than during vertebroplasty [Phillips 2002].

In principle, the cement can escape directly into the greater circulation if either the EVVS or the BS is directly punctured. Furthermore, it is possible that bone marrow enters these veins. The literature describes an increased occurrence of pulmonary embolism after penetration by pedicle screws [Takahashi 2003]. Because of the anatomical situation, the possibility of pulmonary embolism caused by either bone marrow or cement should always be taken into account. The reason for the lower risk of embolism, whether caused by bone marrow or PMMA, during or after balloon kyphoplasty has not been resolved with certainty. The injection of PMMA cement without high pressure plays a decisive role in balloon kyphoplasty [Phillips 2002]; PMMA embolism caused by high-pressure injection of the cement into bone has already been proven to occur in limb surgery [Markel 1999; Orsini 1987]. Furthermore, it is possible that the basivertebral veins are compressed by the balloon and therefore neither fat nor PMMA can pass. A crucial factor regarding the pressure within the whole VVS is the position of the abdomen during the operation.

Compression of the inferior vena cava alone leads to increased blood flow in the VVS via the collateral circulation, and thus to increased risk of embolism [Batson 1940, 1957]. This fact must be taken into account, especially with patients suffering from portal hypertension as a consequence of hepatic cirrhosis. Since cement injection techniques are generally carried out with the patient in an abdominal position, attention should be paid to the intra-abdominal pressure, which must be as low as possible, i.e. the abdomen should be positioned freely during surgery (see Fig. 89, Chapter 11). This means that the venous collateral circulation involving the VVS is reduced to a great extent, and that the blood flows in the caval system. Increased intra-abdominal pressure could theoretically be compensated by increased intrathoracic pressure, preventing collateral circulation and thus increased blood flow through the vertebra [Groen 2004]. However, equalization of the pressure between the two body cavities is impossible without appropriate monitoring during the operation, and such monitoring would be too demanding during surgery. In addition, cardiovascular complications must be taken into account in the case of increased intrathoracic pressure. To conclude, optimal positioning of the patient, relieving the abdomen, is the only remaining efficient prophylaxis for avoiding embolism.

Classification of osteoporotic vertebral fractures

B. Boszczyk

Balloon kyphoplasty is principally suitable for treatment of vertebral fractures that have a localized fragmented zone within the spongiosa and a kyphotic deformity, or for treatment of endplate impression fractures. A precondition for a successful reduction is a healthy vertebral base as a support for the balloon. These criteria are met by fractures of type A1.1 (end plate impression fracture, Fig. 18a), A1.2 (wedge fracture, Fig. 18b, c) and A3.1 (incomplete burst fracture, Fig. 18e–g). According to current knowledge, split fractures (A2), burst fractures (A3.2) and complete burst fractures (A3.3) are not suitable for balloon kyphoplasty, as the splitting component of those fractures cannot be stabilized by the augmentation. However, a complete burst fracture type A3.3 must be distinguished from an osteoporotic collapse of a vertebral body type A1.3 (Fig. 18d) [Magerl 1994]. The latter is suitable for balloon kyphoplasty, as the endplates are hardly fragmented or not fragmented at all, unlike in a complete burst fracture. According to the above criteria for morphology of fractures of the vertebral body, corresponding fractures of group B are also suitable for balloon kyphoplasty, in combination with an internal fixator. This applies to type B1.2 and B2.3 fractures. Precise diagnostics and exact classification of the fracture are indispensable for the successful application of balloon kyphoplasty for those fractures. A combination of computed tomography (CT) and MRI offers the best possible exactness for assessment of osseous and disco-ligamentous injuries.

A criterion that has not yet been examined comprehensively is injury of the adjacent end plate. The classification by Oner provides a graduation of end-plate injuries on the MRI in four degrees of severity, going beyond the conventional classification [Oner 2002]. The first degree merely shows a deformation of the end plate, whereas the second and third degrees each show an isolated injury in the anterior or posterior third of the vertebral body. Injuries reaching throughout the complete endplate are ascribed to the fourth degree. Although no prognostic data on balloon kyphoplasty within this classification system are available, long-term integrity of the intervertebral disc can most probably be assumed in the case of an isolated deformation of the disc or of fissures in the posterior third of the vertebral body.

Reverences

Magerl F, Aebi M, Gertzbein SD, Harms J, Nazarian S (1994) A comprehensive classification of thoracic and lumbar injuries. Eur Spine J 3: 184–201

Oner FC, van Gils APG, Faber AJ, Dhert WJA, Verbout AJ (2002) Some complications of common treatment schemes of thoracolumbar spine fractures can be predicted with magnetic resonance imaging. Spine 27: 629–36

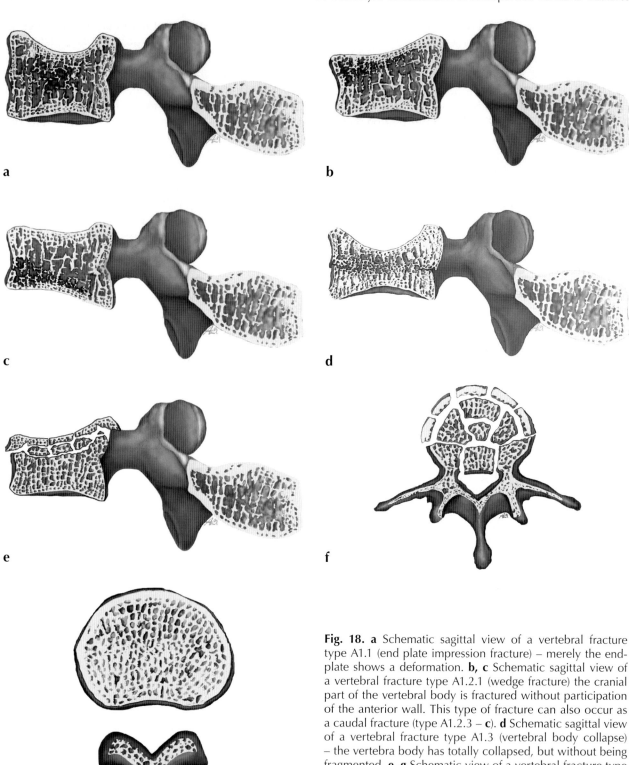

Fig. 18. a Schematic sagittal view of a vertebral fracture type A1.1 (end plate impression fracture) – merely the endplate shows a deformation. **b, c** Schematic sagittal view of a vertebral fracture type A1.2.1 (wedge fracture) the cranial part of the vertebral body is fractured without participation of the anterior wall. This type of fracture can also occur as a caudal fracture (type A1.2.3 – **c**). **d** Schematic sagittal view of a vertebral fracture type A1.3 (vertebral body collapse) – the vertebra body has totally collapsed, but without being fragmented. **e–g** Schematic view of a vertebral fracture type A3.1 (incomplete bursting fracture) – the sagittal view shows the wedge shaped fracture with participation of the anterior wall of the cranial part of the vertebral body; the axial view in the pedicle plane shows the fragmentation of the upper part of the vertebral body (**f**) the axial view beneath the pedicle plane rules out a split fracture (**g**)

Chapter 7

The technique of balloon kyphoplasty

S. Becker

Balloon kyphoplasty is a minimally invasive percutaneous method for stabilizing the spine. The instruments are designed accordingly and together with the inflatable bone tamps (IBT) are described below.

The set of instruments

The basic set of instruments with the bone access tools (Fig. 19) consists of the following:

- 2 Kirschner wires (length 267 mm, blunt and pointed),
- 1 working cannula (osteointroducer). The working cannula is ready to use with a bougie and an additional inlay,
- 1 Jamshidi puncture needle (size s, Chapter 11).

A special set containing a special working cannula (advanced osteointroducer) and an additional drill is available (Fig. 20a, b).

This special working cannula can be used in young patients as well as for hard bones. In principle it differs from the regular working cannula in that it has a 15 mm-long drill at the tip, which makes it easier to introduce the working cannula transpedicularly. It is also advisable to use this instrument in cases under local anesthesia in order to avoid hammering.

The other instruments can be ordered individually packed and opened as required or can be ordered in a package including all necessary tools and balloons to perform a balloon kyphoplasty. In addition, it is possible to use a special curette in order to make a cavity in the bone, so that the balloon can be led in a certain direction, or to enable easier repositioning above the balloon (Fig. 20c, d). The curette can also be used for treating old fractures.

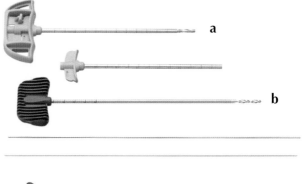

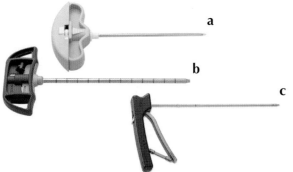

Fig. 19. Basic set of instruments for performing balloon kyphoplasty. **a** Jamshidi puncture needle; **b** Osteointroducer; **c** Kirschner wires

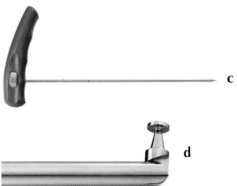

Fig. 20. Set for young patients, hard bones: **a** advanced osteointroducer; **b** drill; **c** curette; **d** tip of the curette

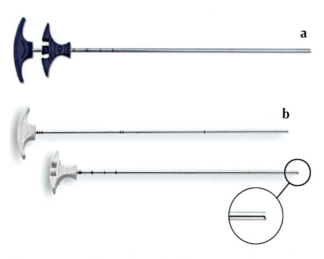

Fig. 21. a Bonefiller with pestle; b biopsy bonefiller

Table 4. Balloon sizes, volume, and maximum pressure

	Length	Maximum content	Maximum pressure
KyphX Xpander®	20 mm	6 ml	400 PSI
KyphX Xpander®	15 mm	4 ml	400 PSI
KyphX Xpander®	10 mm	4 ml	400 PSI
KyphX® Exact™	10 mm	3 ml	300 PSI
	15 mm	4 ml	400 PSI
KyphX® Elevate™	15 mm	4 ml	300 PSI

The following instruments are also necessary: a bone filler (1.5 ml) and a bone biopsy instrument if required (Fig. 21a, b). The bone biopsy instrument looks more or less the same as the bone filler except that it has teeth that taper to a point at the end, which makes the biopsy easier.

The working cannulae, the drill, and the bone filler are marked at intervals of 1 cm so that the depth of penetration into the bone can be followed at any time without x-ray.

The balloon catheter (inflatable) bone tamp and the pressure syringe (Figs. 22, 23)

The balloon (IBT) is the central instrument in balloon kyphoplasty and various types are available.

Conventional balloons (KyphX Xpander®) consist of a balloon, the shaft (length: 293 mm without balloon) and two adapters. One adapter is for attaching the pressure syringe; the other one contains a guide wire. These balloons are available in the sizes 10 mm, 15 mm and 20 mm.

There are also two special balloons especially suited for targeted local reduction of fractures (KyphX® Exact™) or where an large reduction is necessary (KyphX® Elevate™). The shaft length of KyphX® Exact™ is 257 mm and of KyphX® Elevate™ 265 mm, both measured without the balloon.

The capacity for contrast medium of every balloon is limited, as is the maximum applicable pressure. Table 4 gives an overview of the maximum volume and maximum possible pressure for each type of balloon.

A pressure syringe is necessary for filling the balloon. The in-line pressure gauge can indicate the pressure within the balloon in psi (pounds/inch^2) and in atm (atmosphere).

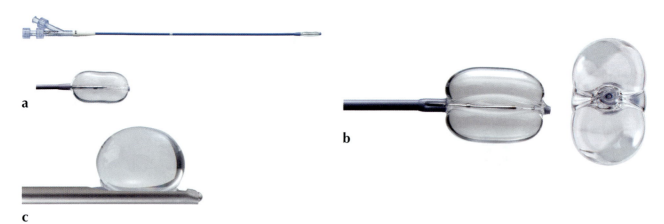

Fig. 22. Balloon catheter. a KyphX Xpander ® 20 mm; b KyphX® Elevate™; c KyphX® Exact™

The technique of balloon kyphoplasty

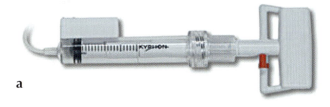

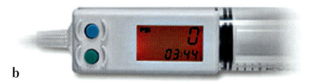

Fig. 23. **a** Pressure syringe, **b** pressure gauge

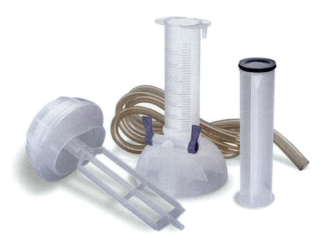

Fig. 24. Cement mixing set

Table 5. Complete set of tools for the performance of balloon kyphoplasty on a lumbar vertebra

---

- 1 basic set of instruments (2 Kirschner wires, 1 handdrill with handle)
- 1 operating cannula (osteointroducer or advanced osteointroducer with a spare inlay)
- 2 x 20 mm kyphoplasty balloons
- 2 pressure syringes
- 2–4 bonefillers
- 1 Jamshidi needle
- 1 scalpel
- 1 Kocher clamp
- 1 hammer
- 1 PMMA cement for balloon kyphoplasty (e.g. KyphX® HV-R)
- 1 dermal suture

Table 5 gives a summary of all the tools and cement needed to carry out a balloon kyphoplasty on a lumbar vertebra.

Anatomical landmarks and image intensifier settings (Figs. 25–27)

Unlike open surgery, where screws are applied transpedicularly at typical points, balloon kyphoplasty differs in that the IBTs must be placed in an optimum position in the middle of the vertebral body in order to achieve best possible reduction of the vertebral fracture without injuring the lateral margins of the vertebral body.

It is thus necessary to define certain landmarks in the image intensifier, which makes operating considerably easier.

It is important to identify the following landmarks on the vertebral body, and set the image converter accordingly: pedicles, spinous process, endplates and the posterior wall.

The pedicles

It is important to know that the pedicles (pedicle rings) visible on the AP image of the image intensifier represent neither the beginning nor the end but the narrowest part of the pedicle. Consequently, it is important that the primary starting point is chosen so that the Jamshidi needle appears to lie outside the pedicle ring on the AP view (Figs. 28, 29). It is also important that the pedicles are reproduced in the upper third of the vertebral body, as this ensures that the vertebral body is not tilted in the sagittal plane.

The spinous process

The spinous process must come to lie centrally on the AP image. It is for the surgeon to decide whether to incline the image intensifier or the operating table until the spinous process lies in the middle. In our experience it is easier to tilt only the image intensifier, particularly if balloon kyphoplasty is being performed on several vertebral bodies. The image intensifier can be tilted faster and more precisely than the operating table.

The endplates and the posterior wall

Both the endplates and the posterior wall must come to lie parallel on the AP and lateral images. Only this can ensure that the IBT lies in a perfect

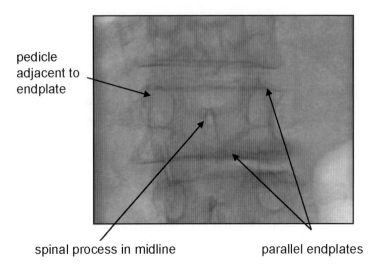

Fig. 25. Spine AP – x-ray with optimal projection

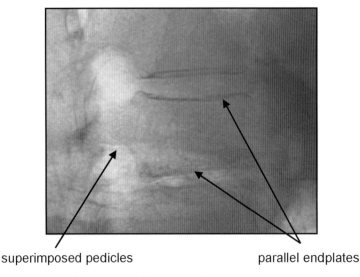

Fig. 26. Spine lat – x-ray with an optimal projection

position and that the vertebra is kyphoplastied properly. A good image of the posterior wall is especially important, as it must be ensured that the working cannula lies ventrally to it in order to avoid leaking of cement.

Special procedures in the case of scoliosis

In a case of scoliotic spine it may well be that an orthograde positioning of the spinous process and the pedicles is impossible. In these cases the image intensifier or the table must be tilted until an orthograde view through the pedicle into the vertebral body is possible (so-called en face or pedicle view,

Fig. 27). If an MRT or CT is available, the inclination of the image intensifier or of the operating table can be set before the operation, making the intra-operative setting much easier.

Starting and end points in lumbar transpedicular operations

Starting point (Figs. 28, 29)

As has been stated above, the starting point, i.e. the point where the Jamshidi needle starts to penetrate into the pedicle, has to be chosen so that the needle

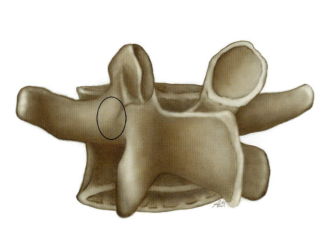 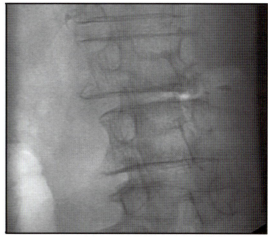

Fig. 27. Diagram and x-ray with an orthograde view through the ipsilateral pedicle (so-called en face or pedicle view image)

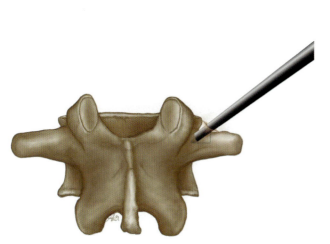 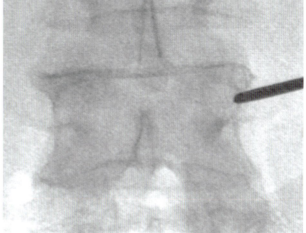

Fig. 28. Starting point of right transpedicular access between 1 and 3 o'clock. The skin incision is 1 cm lateral of this point for L1 to L4, and 2 cm lateral for L5

is apparently outside the pedicle on the AP image. The zones typically chosen in operations of the lumbar spine, including the 11th and 12th thoracic vertebrae, are on the left-hand side 9 to 11 o'clock, and 1 to 3 o'clock on the right-hand side.

End points (Fig. 30)

To make sure that the Jamshidi needle or any other instrument does not perforate the anterior wall of the vertebral body or the spinal canal, end points must be defined. First it is important that the appropriate instrument, in most cases the Kirschner wire, comes to lie approximately 3–4 mm dorsal of the anterior wall, or at the transition point 80%:20% of the vertebral body (Fig. 30a) on the lateral image. The anterior cortical wall cannot always be felt in an osteoporotic vertebra, therefore an end point based on palpation is not safe enough.

The Kirschner wire should not go beyond the center line, i.e. the spinous process on the AP image; an optimum position is achieved if the Kirschner wire touches the transition point 80%:20% of the vertebral body on the lateral image and just touches the spinous process on the AP image (Fig. 30b).

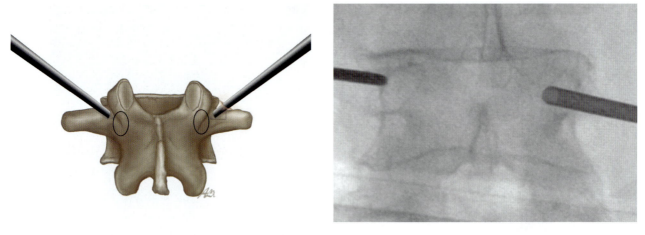

Fig. 29. Starting point of left transpedicular access between 9 and 11 o'clock

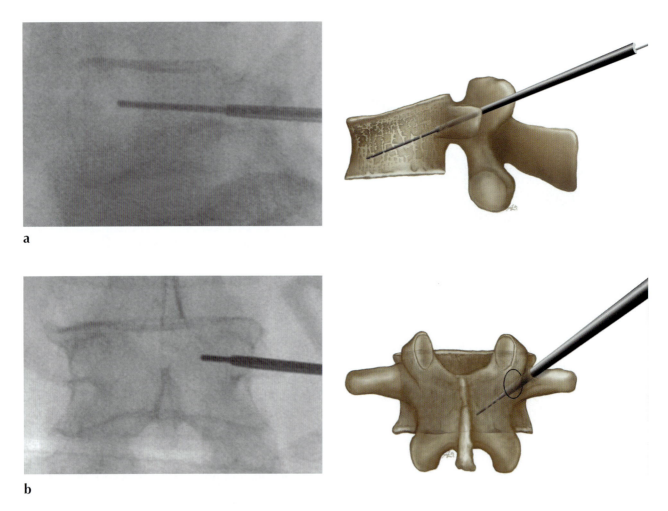

Fig. 30. Ending points for transpedicular access. **a** Ending point of the Kirschner wire on the lateral image approximately 4 mm dorsal of the front edge or at the transition point 80%:20% of the vertebral body. **b** Ending point of the Kirschner wire on the AP image, convergence towards the centre line, which however should not be crossed

Starting and end points in thoracic extrapedicular operations (Fig. 31)

Although the end point for extrapedicular access into the thoracic spine is the same as the end point for transpedicular access, the starting point is different. Cranial of Th10 a transpedicular access is not possible any more because of the size and form of the vertebrae, which do not allow the balloon to be positioned in an optimum way. When accessing extrapedicularly, the first bone contact is the craniodorsal corner of the end plate, because of the anatomical situation (Fig. 31a), and not the pedicle as in transpedicular access. The Jamshidi needle therefore has to be orientated towards the respective cranial corner of the vertebral body as a starting point on the AP image (Fig. 31b). The optimum situation is that, when touching the corner, the posterior wall has already been reached (more detailed instructions are in the chapter on carrying out balloon kyphoplasty). As already mentioned, the end point of the Kirschner wire or the balloon is the

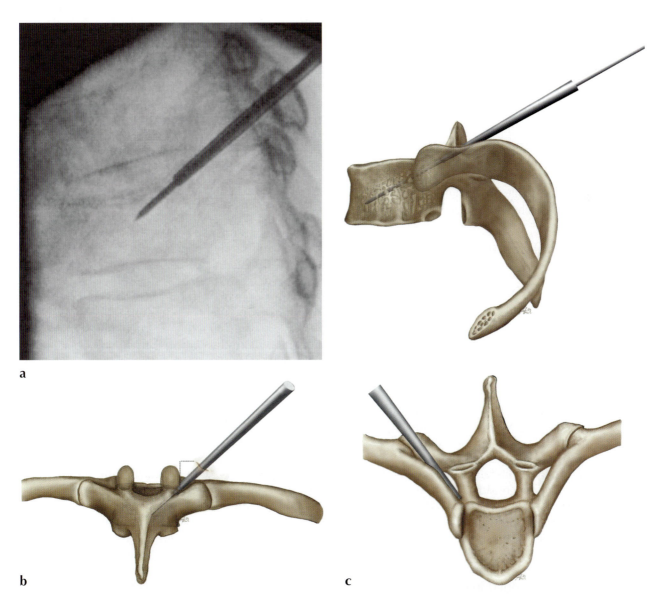

Fig. 31. Starting/ending points of extrapedicular access, **a** analogue to Fig. 29. **b** Ending point analogue to Fig. 30b, note that the skin incision is carried out 1 cm lateral and 2 cm cranially of the starting point which is located on the lateral upper vertebral wall. **c** Axial presentation of the perforation point of the trailing edge of the vertebral body

same as in transpedicular access, i.e. the maximum is the 80% : 20% limitation on the lateral image and the center line on the AP image (Fig. 31a, b).

Preparation and positioning of the patient

From our own experience we recommend giving patients a laxative on the day preceding the operation. This ensures optimum presentation of the spine in the image intensifier without the overlapping of bowel gas, which could have a negative influence on an already poor image of an osteoporotic spine. Because of the anatomical situation of the venous plexus surrounding the vertebra (Figs. 16, 17, Chapter 6), the patient should be placed in a prone position so that only the thorax and pelvis rest on the table and the abdomen hangs free. This allows closed reduction of a fracture and prevents increased bloodflow through the vertebra, which could encourage cement or fat embolism. One or two image intensifiers, depending on the local situation, may be used during the operation; we routinely operate using only one image intensifier which can be oriented easily according to the demands.

Performing balloon kyphoplasty

The impact of positioning versus balloon kyphoplasty on restoration of vertebral height

In trauma management, closed reduction of a vertebral facture has been performed for decades. The widely reported ligamentotaxis of the anterior and posterior longitudinal ligaments helps to restore vertebral congruity. The question therefore arises of whether postoperative gain in vertebral height is due to the balloon or simply to positioning the patient in a prone position on the table (Fig. 32, see also figures in osteonecrosis chapter).

It is reported in the literature that balloon kyphoplasty significantly increases vertebral height and reduces kyphosis [Ledlie 2003; Lieberman 2001; Phillips 2003], but there are also reports of significant reduction of kyphosis by positioning alone [Faciszewski 2002; McKiernan 2003]. The significant loss of vertebral height after deflation of the balloon has been reported in comparison with vertebral height with the balloon in situ; nevertheless, overall kyphosis and correction of vertebral height was still significantly better after balloon kyphoplas-

ty than after positioning [Voggenreiter 2005]. However, those studies did not include osteonecrotic fractures, where total collapse of the vertebra may cause greater instability of the vertebral bodies and therefore theoretically greater collapse of the vertebral body after removal of the balloons (see chapter on osteonecrosis).

We therefore analyzed the effects of positioning and balloon kyphoplasty in patients with osteonecrotic fractures (same patient group as in the osteonecrosis chapter). The difference between closed reduction in the OR and restoration of postoperative height with balloon kyphoplasty is shown in Table 6.

In contrast to other studies, our results showed no significant difference between the postoperative height correction of the vertebral body and the primary correction gained by positioning [Voggenreiter 2005], possibly a consequence of the greater dynamic instability in osteonecrotic fractures. Nevertheless, the feared loss of reduction after removal of the balloon did not occur. Because of the limited number of patients, we performed detailed statistical analysis including partial eta^2 values and found a tendency to correction of the mid-vertebral height only in the group with osteonecrosis (eta^2 0.274).

In conclusion, we found that closed reduction alone significantly reduces vertebral height in patients with osteonecrosis and that the balloon may help to increase the mid-vertebral height.

In our opinion, closed reduction by positioning osteonecrosis patients on the OR table allows good reduction of the fracture, particularly in these patients in whom the best result can still be achieved with balloon kyphoplasty.

Anesthesiological preparation

Balloon kyphoplasty can be performed under general or local anesthesia. We prefer general anesthesia for multiple levels. Reasons for carrying out balloon kyphoplasty under local anesthesia could be that the method is preferred by the surgeon, or that general anesthesia is contraindicated, or the medical history of the patient rules out general anesthesia. In this case however, it should be ensured that the patient also receives a sedative. Local anesthesia should anesthetize the pedicle, i.e. a depot of the local anesthetic should be brought directly at the starting point into the pedicle. The correct starting point is often missed at first, therefore it is advisable to apply the anesthetic generously to the pedicle. Further-

Table 6. Percentage of restored vertebral height (*AH* anterior height, *MH* middle height, *PH* posterior height) during closed reduction and after balloon kyphoplasty (*ON* osteonecrosis, *VP* vertebra plana without osteonecrosis)

	AH – mean	MH – mean	PH – mean
ON Group (n = 8) – after closed reduction	72.71 SD 7.13	56.42 SD 15.84	74.28 SD 9.96
ON Group – after balloon kyphoplasty	75.71 SD 12.04	71.46 SD 15.32	82.67 SD 11.87
p/eta²	0.49/0.081	0.183/0.274	0.26/0.200
VP Group (n = 7) – after closed reduction	48.83 SD 25.67	53.00 SD 25.75	72.00 SD 21.53
VP Group – after balloon kyphoplasty	58.54 SD 17.91	53.26 SD 14.27	75.72 SD 12.01
p/eta²	0.50/0.094	0.995/0.000	0.78/0.017

more, it can also be necessary to introduce a depot of local anesthetic into the vertebra itself before inflating the balloon, as this can be painful.

Lumbar transpedicular access

Transpedicular access is suitable for kyphoplasting vertebrae Th10 to L5. Depending on the size of the patient and of the pedicles, it may be that extrapedicular access must be chosen in the area of Th10.

After positioning the patient in the appropriate manner, the image intensifier should be set for an AP image, and the typical point for penetration into the pedicle should be marked on the surface of the skin. Because of the convergence of the pedicles, the incision in the area of Th12 to L4 should be

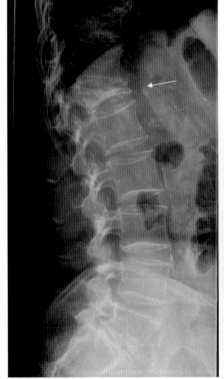
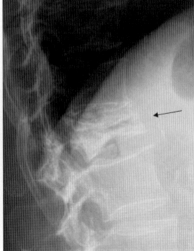

Fig. 32. Female, 66 years, spontaneous onset of pain 4 weeks ago, osteoporotic fracture Th12 with suspicion of osteonecrosis (**a**). By positioning in the X-ray department, the kyphotic angle could be reduced from 32° (**a**) to 21° (**b**). The vertebra clearly shows signs of osteonecrosis

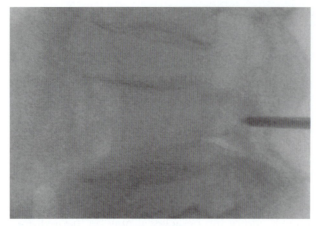
a

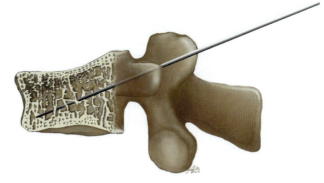
b

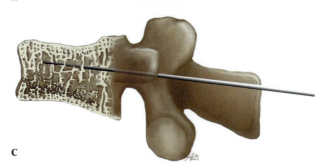
c

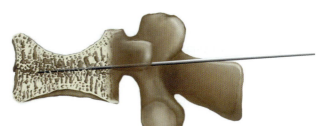
d

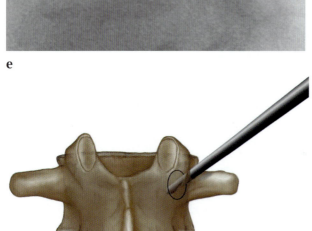
e

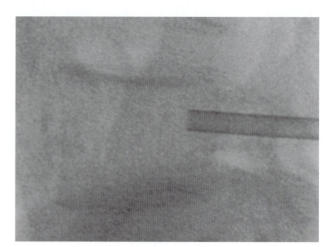
f

The technique of balloon kyphoplasty

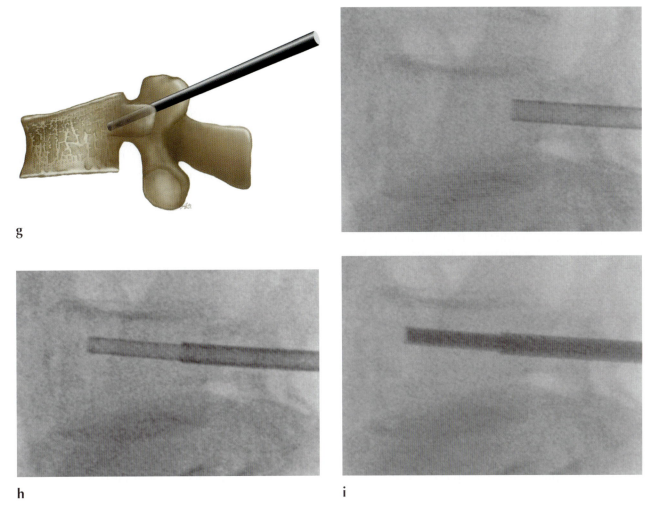

Fig. 33. Introduction of the Jamshidi needle and the operating cannula (osteointroducer). **a** Starting point of the Jamshidi needle on the lateral view. **b–d** The cranial-caudal orientation of the Jamshidi needle has to be adapted according to the type of fracture. **b** Fracture type A1.2.1. **c** Fracture type A1.2.3. **d** Fracture type A1.3. **e** Ending point of the Jamshidi needle with a slight perforation of the posterior wall on the lateral view. **f** Ending point of the Jamshidi needle on the AP view. The medial limitation of the pedicle ring should not be exceeded. **g** Ending point of the operating cannula at least 2–3 mm ventrally of the posterior wall of the vertebral body. **h** Biopsy with bonefiller. **i** Preparing the cannula for the balloon

1 cm lateral of the typical starting point into the pedicle (Figs. 28, 29). An exact skin incision is very important as this determines proper convergence of the Jamshidi needle towards the pedicle and also ensures that the surrounding muscular and soft tissues do not divert the Jamshidi needle during the control image. With obese patients it is advisable to hold the Jamshidi needle with an instrument during the image intensifier control.

After situating the Jamshidi needle properly at the starting point into the pedicle on the AP image, the pedicle should be slightly perforated and the Jamshidi needle advanced a few millimeters into the pedicle.

A lateral image is then taken with the image intensifier (Fig. 33a). This enables orientation of the Jamshidi needle, depending on the kind of fracture. In normal wedge-shaped vertebrae it is recommended that the Jamshidi needle is aligned parallel to the deck plate, in concave fractures in the middle, and in fractures of the basal lamina in the direction of the basal lamina (Fig. 33b–d). Normally, it should now be possible to introduce the Jamshidi needle without problems transpedicularly in the already pre-determined direction up to the posterior wall, purely by palpation and without an image intensifier control. The first osseous resistance is where the tip of the Jamshidi needle has reached the posterior wall (Fig. 33e). Contrary to common belief, the pedicle is not continuously open into the vertebra. As a result of embryonic development, the posterior wall is usually readily palpable even in the transpedicular approach. In practical terms this means, bearing in mind the radiological protection of the patient and the operation team, that for transpedicular introduction of the Jamshidi needle there is no necessity for an image intensifier control before a hard resistance is felt. The optimum situation is that when this hard resistance is felt, the needle has already reached the posterior wall. If this is not the case, the AP and lateral positions have to be corrected accordingly. It is sufficient to perforate the posterior wall only 1–2 mm with the Jamshidi needle. If the needle is positioned in an optimum way, it should not exceed the medial limitation of the pedicle on the AP image (Fig. 33f). At this point it is still easy to correct the position of the Kirschner wire, which, unlike the working cannula, causes much less damage to the posterior wall in case of misplacement (Fig. 36). Now the blunt Kirschner wire is advanced through the Jamshidi needle; the pointed Kirschner wire which is also delivered in the balloon kyphoplasty set is more suited for young patients with hard bone. The Kirschner wire allows simulation of the end point of the balloon, as described above (Fig. 30a, b). It is important to record the end position of the Kirschner wire on both AP and lateral images and, in case it lies too medial or too lateral, to correct the position either by inserting the Jamshidi needle anew or, as we do in our clinic, by changing the orientation of the working cannula.

Once the Kirschner wire has been brought into the proper position the Jamshidi needle can be removed and the working cannula introduced (the regular working cannula for normal osteoporotic fractures or the advanced osteointroducer for young patients). It must be ensured, particularly in the case of osteoporosis or of correction of the angle of the working cannula that the Kirschner wire is pulled backwards of the vertebral body to avoid anterior perforation during working channel insertion.

The working cannula is driven in transpedicularly until it comes to lie about 3 mm ventrally of the posterior wall of the vertebra (Fig. 33g). This ensures

that the working cannula is fixed in the posterior wall and that leakage of cement is impossible.

It is important that once the working cannula has been brought into the posterior wall its position should not be changed again. If the cannula is removed or moved accidentally, there is a risk of creating a second hole in the posterior wall when positioning it anew. If the pedicle has been perforated at the transition point of the pedicle to the posterior wall with the first hole, there is a high risk of cement leaking into the spinal canal. Therefore the working cannula should not be removed from the posterior wall of the vertebra, even if it is not in a 100% optimal position.

At this stage a transpedicular biopsy can be taken, either with the biopsy instrument or with the bone filler (Fig. 33h). If the vertebral body is very hard it may be necessary to drill a canal for the balloon with a hand-drill instead of carrying out the biopsy. When taking the biopsy, care should be taken not to perforate the anterior wall.

After carrying out the biopsy or the drilling, the bone canal must be smoothed by repeatedly bringing in a bone filler which is equipped with a pestle. This is to avoid pointed edges in the bone, as these could perforate the balloon when it is being inflated (Fig. 33i).

After smoothing the canal in the vertebral body, a balloon chosen according to the size of the vertebral body can be introduced. Both balloons should be introduced and inflated simultaneously. As an optimum, the balloon should come to lie in the middle of the vertebral body and with both markings outside the working cannula (Fig. 34). The pressure syringe is then brought into the 0 ml position by applying pressure to the handle. The pressure gauge is turned on with the green button on the LCD box, and then the units can be changed from atm to psi with the blue button (Fig. 23b). It is advisable to carry out the balloon kyphoplasty using the psi scale as this is divided into smaller units and is thus more sensitive. Now, by turning the handle 360 degrees clockwise for each 0.5 ml, the contrast medium can be brought into the balloon.

Note: It is advisable to use an iodine contrast medium as visualization in the image intensifier is much better. However, if the patient suffers from iodine allergy it is advisable to add undiluted gadolinium to the balloon.

The balloon should be inflated with a pressure of approx. 50 psi. After that the guide wire (Fig. 22) may be removed. This ensures that the balloon

The technique of balloon kyphoplasty

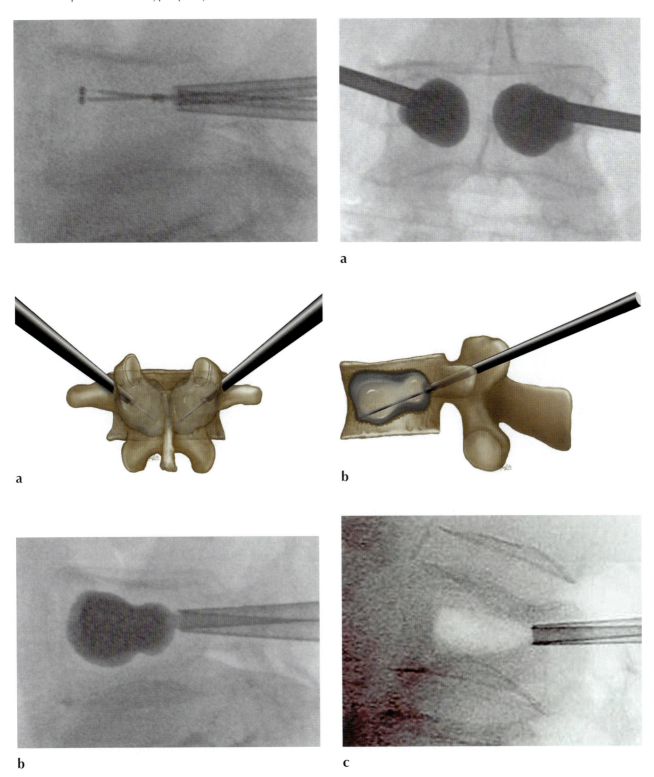

Fig. 34. Non-inflated balloons in the vertebra, both markings of the balloons must lie outside of the operating cannula. **a, b** Ending points of the balloons, the balloons should not perforate any cortical substance, neither on the AP (**a**), nor on the lateral (**b**) view. **c** The removal of the balloons leaves an extensive cavity in the vertebra

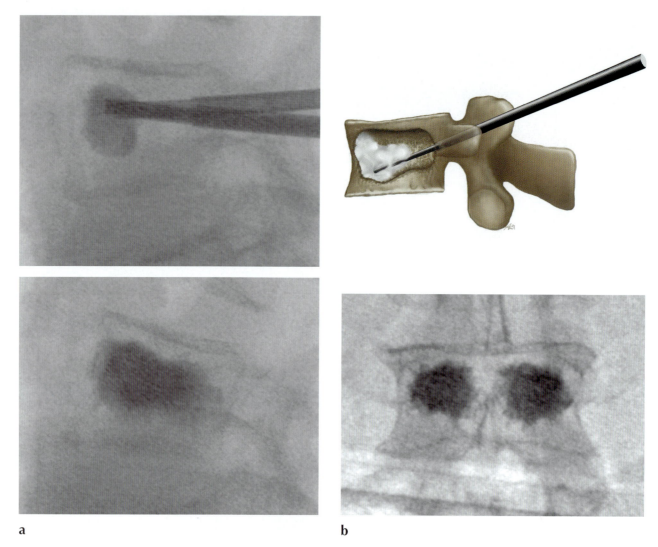

Fig. 35. Retrograde filling of the vertebral body with bonefiller; it has to be kept in position during the filling process. **a, b** Filling the vertebral body with a sufficient amount of cement (here 3 ml on both sides), which is firmly connected with the spongiosa

keeps its original form and situation. The reason for removing the guide wire is to allow the balloon to expand without hindrance in the direction of the lowest bone resistance. This maneuver is not necessary when using the Exact or the Elevator balloon. After removing the guide wire the balloon can be inflated to the required size. It is advisable to carry out an AP image intensifier control after bringing 1 ml of contrast medium into the balloon in order to ensure that neither balloon perforates the cortical substance laterally.

The inflation of the balloon is continued until either the maximum amount of contrast medium has been introduced, the maximum pressure within the balloon has been reached (see Table 4), or the endplates or the lateral vertebral body walls are touched (Fig. 34a, b). The volume of medium brought into the balloon may be determined from the graduation marks on the pressure syringe; the amount of cement may be deduced from the volume of the balloon. Removal of the balloons often leaves a clearly visible cavity in the vertebra (Fig. 34c).

The cement can now be introduced into the vertebral body. It is advisable to keep the balloons within the vertebral body until the cement has reached the appropriate viscosity (Fig. 41). This en-

The technique of balloon kyphoplasty

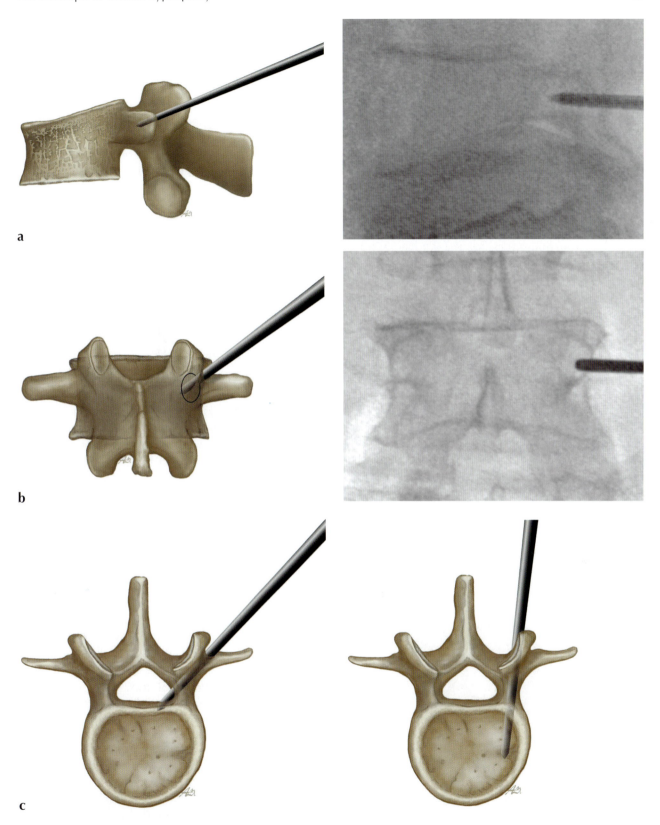

Fig. 36. Indications of potential incorrect positions (see text). **a** Proper position of the Jamshidi needle on the lateral view; **b** proper position of the Jamshidi needle on the AP view; **c** medial perforation; **d** operating cannula too lateral

sures that no additional blood or fat is pressed into the blood circulation as the result of injecting the cement. The balloons must be emptied completely by squeezing the handle and drawing it back. It is advisable to hold the working cannula with one hand while withdrawing the balloon so that it cannot be dislocated from the pedicle.

If this does happen, the working cannula should calmly be applied to the vertebra body again, according to the above procedure. It is better to discard a packet of cement than to risk having the working cannula lying in the wrong position.

After the removal of the balloons, the bone fillers must be brought into the working cannula. At this point the graduation marks are helpful (Fig. 21). The first thick graduation line on the bone filler indicates that it has not yet left the working cannula. The bone filler is marked with one, two or three further lines which correspond to the depth of its penetration into the vertebral body after leaving the working cannula. It is usually safe to drive the bone filler two lines deep into the vertebral body, even without an image intensifier control.

The bone filler should be introduced at least two graduation lines deep into the vertebral body. It is advisable to bring in both bone fillers and, under continuous image intensifier control, to first fill one side then the other with cement. This ensures that in case of cement leakage, it can be related to a specific side.

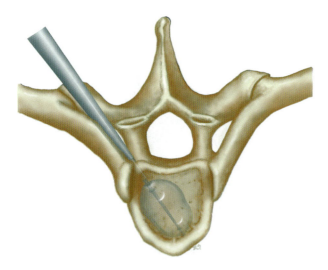

Fig. 37. Schematic axial view of a transcostovertebrally introduced balloon kyphoplasty balloon. Increased convergence allows a central position of each individual balloon

The bone filler should be left in its anterior position to ensure retrograde homogeneous filling of the vertebral body (Fig. 35). The maximum amount of cement usually corresponds with the maximum volume in the balloon, but in cases where additional filling is necessary, an additional 0.5 ml of cement can be applied per pedicle; however, it is necessary to monitor this additional filling closely.

After the vertebral body has been filled with the required quantity of cement on both sides, both bone fillers should be drawn back to the first line in order to avoid the cement being pulled out along with the bone filler into the pedicle. The bone filler should be left in this position in the bone until the cement has hardened.

A final AP and lateral image completes the intraoperative documentation (Fig. 35a, b).

Further special techniques, such as the egg shell technique, are explained in Chapter 9.

Extrapedicular access

In the extrapedicular approach the incision of the skin is in a different place from that in the transpedicular approach (Fig. 31b). The optimal incision of the skin is 1 cm lateral and 2 cm proximal of the starting point, i.e. of the lateral endplate corner. It should then be possible to introduce the Jamshidi needle into the vertebral body between the rib and the transverse process without resistance up to the posterior wall (Fig. 31a, c). However, because of the anatomical situation, it is possible that the canal between the rib and the transverse process is so narrow that the Jamshidi needle cannot be driven in without using a hammer. The same applies for facet joint arthritis. This is not dangerous if, with an optimal incision, the needle is led towards the corner of the vertebral body on the AP image. Under all circumstances the Jamshidi needle must not be introduced into the vertebral body below the pedicle on the lateral x-ray, because the nerve root and segmental vessels run here.

Extrapedicular access requires a little more practice than transpedicular access; however, it is just as safe as transpedicular access if the needle is directed at the lateral vertebral corner.

After perforating the posterior wall of the vertebra with the Jamshidi needle by 1 to 2 mm, the introduction of the Kirschner wire, the following of image intensifier controls and the further steps of the operation should be performed according to the transpedicular approach.

The technique of balloon kyphoplasty

In the extrapedicular approach, the Kirschner wire may cross the spinous process on the AP image. This happens if the Kirschner wire or the Jamshidi needle converge too much, and the balloon is brought too far towards the center of the vertebral body (Fig. 37). This is not as important here as it is in transpedicular access, as the entrance point is lateral of the pedicle anyway (Fig. 31c). However, it could prove impossible to introduce the second balloon; in this case we leave the primary balloon in situ and perform balloon kyphoplasty with only one balloon.

Malpositioning of the working cannula
(Figs. 36, 37)

In principle, lateral and medial malpositions of the osteointroducer have to be avoided because there is a danger of perforating the pedicle or the lateral vertebral body wall. It is therefore necessary to detect any danger of malpositioning immediately after introducing the Jamshidi needle. If wrong positioning is suspected, an image-intensifier image should be made in the AP view when the Jamshidi needle has approximately reached the middle of the pedicle on the lateral image (Fig. 36a). In ideal positioning, the tip of the needle should lie approximately in the middle of the pedicle (Fig. 36b) on the AP image; however, if the needle has already reached the medial limitation of the pedicle ring (Fig. 33f) there is a danger of perforating the pedicle medially (Fig. 36c). If, however, on the AP image the needle is close to the starting point, the working cannula (osteointroducer) is most likely to lie too far laterally (Fig. 36d). A too lateral position does not always have to be corrected, though in this case care has to be taken when inflating the balloon, in order not to perforate the lateral vertebral body wall.

There is also the danger of injuring the surrounding anatomical structures when accessing extrapedicularly (Fig. 38a, b). If the Jamshidi needle enters too far sagittally it can injure the pleura and the lungs, and a ventral perforation can injure the big thoracic vessels. An entrance below the pedicle or a cranial orientation endangers the spinal nerves

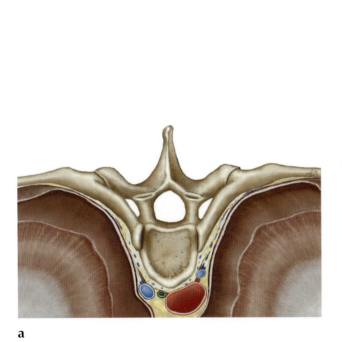
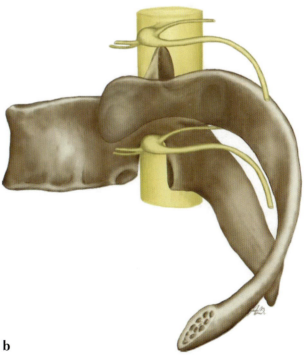

Fig. 38. Anatomy of the middle thoracic spine. **a** Note the proximity of the vertebra to the big thoracic vessels, to the pleura and to the lungs. **b** An introduction of the Jamshidi needle beneath the pedicle endangers the corresponding spinal nerves

and the intercostal vessels. Therefore it is absolutely necessary to make an exact skin incision and to orientate the needle exactly towards the upper lateral limitation of the vertebral body.

References

Faciszewski T, McKiernan F (2002) Calling all vertebral fractures classification of vertebral compression fractures: a consensus for comparison of treatment and outcome. J Bone Miner Res 17(2): 185–91

Ledlie JT, Renfro M (2003) Balloon kyphoplasty: one-year outcomes in vertebral body height restoration, chronic pain and activity levels. J Neurosurg Spine 98 [1 Suppl]: 36–42

Lieberman IH, Dudeney S, Reinhardt MK, Bell G (2001) Initial outcome and efficacy of kyphoplasty in the treatment of painful osteoporotic vertebral compression fractures. Spine 26(14): 1631–8

McKiernan F, Jensen R, Faciszewski T (2003) The dynamic mobility of vertebral compression fractures. J Bone & Mineral Res b 18: 24–9

Phillips FM, Ho E, Campbell-Hupp M, McNally T, Todd Wetzel F, Gupta P (2003) Early radiographic and clinical results of balloon kyphoplasty for the treatment of osteoporotic vertebral compression fractures. Spine 28(19): 2260–5

Voggenreiter G (2005) Balloon kyphoplasty is effective in deformity correction of osteoporotic vertebral compression fractures. Spine 30(24): 2806–12

High thoracic approach

B. Boszczyk

The transpedicular route has become popular for VP under fluoroscopic guidance [Lin 2001]. The KP working cannula however, through which the balloon is passed, has a large diameter of 4,2 mm, which is only inconsistently suitable for pedicles of the upper thoracic vertebrae which have a reported width of 2,5–7 mm (average 4,5–5 mm) between T4–T6 [Zindrick 1987]. These vertebrae consistently have the most slender pedicles of the thoracic spine [McLain 2002; Tan 2004; Zindrick 1987] and the percentage of vertebrae with a pedicle width of less than 4,5 mm is given as 33% for T4, 25% for T5 and 17% for T6 in Caucasians [McLain 2002]. In Asian populations a transpedicular route for KP may be unsuitable altogether at certain levels (average width of ~4 mm at T4–T6 in Singaporean Chinese [Tan 2004]). The strong sagittal alignment of upper thoracic pedicles and the relatively small size of the vertebral bodies further increase the difficulty of achieving sufficient tool convergence for central balloon placement. While needle placement in VP is somewhat less crucial for the success of the procedure, as cement flow will often distribute sufficiently from an excentric placement, the desired effect of vertebral body height increase in KP is dependent upon relatively central expansion of the balloon under the endplate.

The patient is positioned prone on cushions and the affected vertebral body is localised with biplanar fluoroscopy. For high thoracic procedures it is advisable to keep the arms adducted next to the body with a bolster placed under the sternum, to allow the shoulders to drop forward and out of the path of the fluoroscopy beam. The anterior-posterior (ap) view is adjusted with the spinous process of the targeted vertebral body in the exact midline, endplates parallel and pedicles placed symmetrically in the upper lateral quadrant of the projection of the vertebral body. The lateral (lat) view is adjusted with pedicles superimposed, endplates parallel and the posterior wall aligned with a single contour. After draping, the costal angle associated with the targeted vertebral body is localised in the ap view and a transverse stab incision is placed immediately superior to its cranial border. A bone biopsy needle is introduced from craniolateral towards the costovertebral joint. Contact is made with the neck of the rib or the transverse process. Ideally, the needle is then slid along the neck of the rib, passing under the transverse process and penetrating the ligament complex of the costovertebral joint until the lateral pedicle wall is reached (Fig. 39a–c). In the fluoroscopic ap view the tip of the needle should be projected at the craniolateral border of the targeted pedicle cortex. In the corresponding lat view, the tip of the needle should be projected between the superior and inferior border of the pedicle, anterior to the facet joints and close to the base of the pedicle. A projection of the tip of the needle posterior to the facet joint indicates placement on the transverse process – in this case a more cranial starting point should enable the needle to pass under the transverse process along the neck of the rib. Once the needle is correctly placed (Fig. 39), it is tapped through the lateral pedicle cortex. Before passing the posterior vertebral wall into the vertebral body in the lat view, the tip of the needle should be verified within the pedicle ring on the ap view. Only after having passed the posterior vertebral wall on the lat view may the tip of the needle cross the medial pedicle wall in the ap view. Strict adherence to these landmarks is mandatory for the avoidance of spinal perforation. A guide wire is now placed through the biopsy needle, which serves to direct the KP working cannula along the same track. The KP balloon is then placed convergently into the vertebral body, close to the anterior cortex (Fig. 40). Balloon inflation and cement augmentation do not differ from the transpedicular technique [Boszczyk 2005]. After cement augmentation has been completed, the working cannula is withdrawn and the stab incision is closed with a single suture. The instillation of 2 ml of local anaesthetic into the cannula, as it is withdrawn, can help alleviate postoperative discomfort from mechanical irritation of the costovertebral joint.

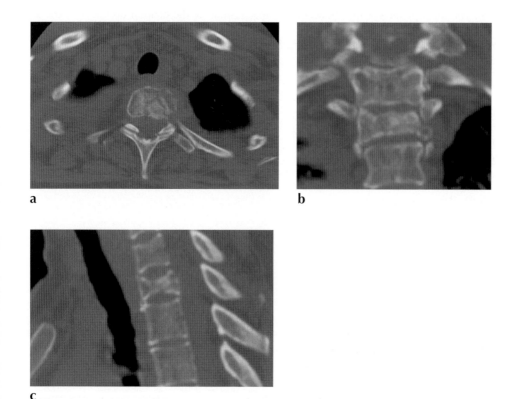

Fig. 39. Pathological fracture of T2 with metastasis of a cervix carcinoma of a 52-year-old patient with a disseminated metastasis [Boszczyk et al. 2005]. The preoperative computer tomography shows the vertebral collapse on the transversal (**a**), frontal (**b**), and sagittal (**c**) reconstruction

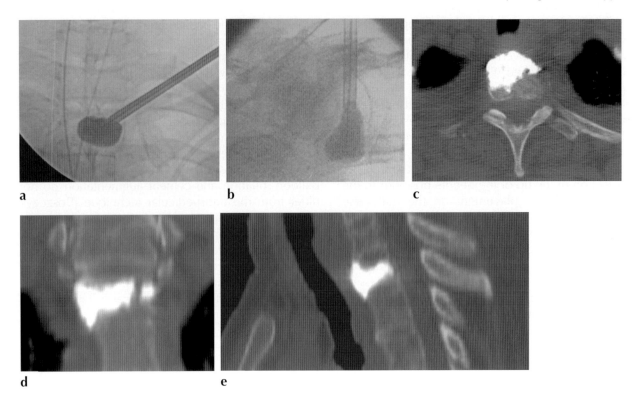

Fig. 40. Same patient as in Fig. 38. The intraoperative X-ray shows the central position of the balloon on the AP view (**a**) and on the lateral view. The view of the anterior wall is hindered by an overlapping of the shoulder girdle (**b**). The postoperative computed tomography on a transversal (**c**), frontal (**d**), and sagittal (**e**) view documents the proper position of the applied PMMA

References

Boszczyk BM, Bierschneider M, Hauck S, Beisse R, Potulski M, Jaksche H (2005) Transcostovertebral kyphoplasty of the mid- and high-thoracic spine. Eur Spine J 14(10): 992–9

Lin DD, Gailloud P, Murphy KJ (2001) Percutaneous vertebroplasty in benign and malignant disease. Neurosurgery Quarterly 11: 290–301

McLain RF, Ferrera L, Kabins M (2002) Pedicle morphology in the upper thoracic spine. Spine 27: 2467–71

Tan SH, Teo EC, Chua HC (2004) Quantitative three-dimensional anatomy of cervical, thoracic and lumbar vertebrae of Chinese Singaporeans. Eur Spine J 13: 137–46

Zindrick MR, Wiltse LL, Doornik A, Widell EH, Knight GW, Patwardhan AG, Thomas JC, Rothman SL, Fields BT (1987) Analysis of the morphometric characteristics of the thoracic and lumbar pedicles. Spine 12: 160–6

Instructions for preparation of the cement

S. Becker

Cement leakage has to be avoided in all spinal percutaneous augmentation methods. The risk of leakage is greater the more liquid the cement, i.e. the lower its viscosity, therefore the cement used in kyphoplasty has to have a certain consistency. We use the PMMA cement KyphX® HV-R (Kyphon, Sunnyvale, USA) for balloon kyphoplastic surgery. The instructions given in the following refer to this cement; if other cements are used, the corresponding instructions given by the manufacturers should be observed.

Depending on the level of training and experience of the surgeon, preparation of the cement can be carried out in such a manner that it has the optimal consistency precisely when all instruments have been brought in into the vertebral body, and the vertebral body has been restored by the kyphoplasty balloons. Beginners are advised to mix the cement a little later, and to first calmly restore the vertebra, instead of being concerned about early hardening of the cement and thus possibly ignoring certain safety guidelines.

The cement is mixed from two compounds in the usual manner, and can be applied directly to the bone filler device. A bone filler contains 1.5 ml of cement; the total amount of the cement to be applied is determined by the maximum volume of the kyphoplasty balloon. The cement has the right consistency as soon as it no longer drips from the syringe or the bone filler (Fig. 41). For loading bone fillers, it has proven to be practical to fill a 2 ml syringe for each device. It is easier to use a 2 ml syringe, especially for refilling a bone filler, than using a syringe with a larger volume. Another tip for the consistency of the cement: it has optimal con-

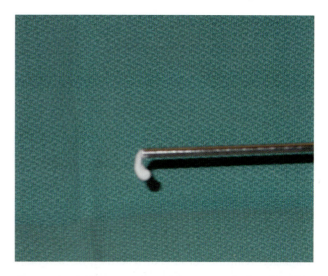

Fig. 41. Optimal consistency of the cement before filling the cavity with the bonefiller

sistency to be brought into the vertebral body when it is like chewing gum and no longer sticks to the operation glove.

The cement usually reaches optimal consistency 8–9 minutes after mixing, and can be applied within the next 6 minutes. After that the cement becomes so hard that it cannot be brought into the bone through the bone filler, and after a total of 19 to 20 minutes the cement (KyphX® HV-R) has reached its final hardness.

If required, a KyphX® cement-mixing instrument can be used to mix the cement (Fig. 24); this allows several bone fillers to be loaded, and at the same time the exposure of the operation team to cement monomers and solvents is reduced. However, if the mixer is used, the cement hardening time is reduced and therefore application time limited.

Radiation exposure

B. Boszczyk and M. Bierschneider

Exposure time (ET) is almost always longer in the lat view due to the monitoring of PMMA injection, which relies heavily on the lat view for recognising even minimal epidural or paravertebral venous leakage. In an investigation on 60 patients an average ET_{lat} of 2,2 min was required in cases treated for single levels [Boszczyk 2006] (Fig. 42). When treating multiple level cases, the ET_{lat} per level was reduced to 1,7 min per level. This finding is due to the considerable imaging overlap between adjacent levels. Up to three adjacent vertebrae can ideally be visualised with the same C-arm setting, occasionally allowing simultaneous PMMA injection.

The addition of ET_{ap} and ET_{lat} to a total ET per treated level or case is not rational from a dosimetrical standpoint as they relate to different projections. Nevertheless, total ET per level provides the clinician with a rough guideline as to the amount of radiation that is "used" and may allow an – acknowledgeably unscientific – comparison between different operative set-ups and techniques. With this restriction in mind, average total ET per level in single fracture cases was 3,8 min (range 1,1–6,6 min). In multiple level cases, the average total ET per level was 2,8 min (range 1,1–4,5 min). Corresponding total ET per level in multiple level VP cases (average 4,25 vertebrae per session) by Harstall et al. [2004] was slightly lower with 2,2 min. This may reflect the greater technical demand of KP over VP during tool introduction and balloon inflation. Although the risk/benefit ratio of the techniques will need to be clarified through comparative studies, it is unlikely that such a minor difference in ET will be found to be of any clinical significance.

The calculated entrance skin dose (ESD) values of the above patients 3 shows that the 2 Gy threshold to early transient erythema [Wagner 1994] was not reached in either plane. Correspondingly, no signs of erythema developed in any of the patients. ESD_{ap} was well within the safety limit with an average of 0,23 Gy and even the maximum value only reaching 0,86 Gy. ESD_{lat} is of greater concern, as the average value reached 0,68 Gy and the maximum value rose to 1,43 Gy. The latter value was obtained in a patient treated for two adjacent vertebral fractures (L1, L2) with an ET_{lat} of 3,6 minutes. In cases that are difficult to visualise (e.g. pre-existing scoliosis) or that require continuous live fluoroscopy during PMMA injection due to complex pathology (e.g. posterior wall disruption or osteolysis) it is conceivable that ET_{lat} could reach levels of concern. The use of a larger C-arm, would hereby markedly reduce ESD, as skin exposure drops along an inverse second order function with increased skin to focus distance.

Effective dose (E) values were found to reach an average of 4,28 mSv. The lifetime risk of developing a cancer after a single KP procedure is theoretically

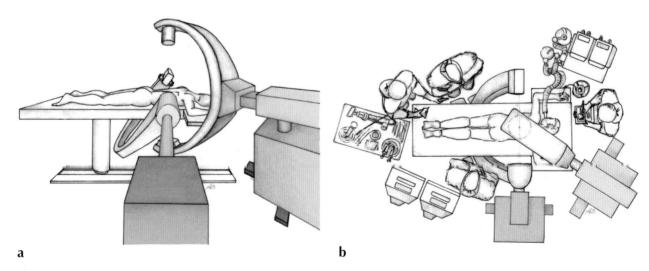

Fig. 42. Drawing of the image intensifier setting for percutaneous balloon kyphoplasty with biplanar screening; view from the side (**a**) view from above (**b**). Surgeon and assistant are standing to the side of the patient, the anesthesist is at the head end, and the instruments are handed from the foot

increased by 0,02–0,06%. These values are to be seen in relation to a baseline of 20–25% cause of death from cancer in the Western European population. This 20–25% lifetime risk of developing a fatal cancer is therefore theoretically increased by 0,02% for the mean E value of 4,28 mSv and by 0,05% for the maximum E value of 10,14 mSv after a single KP procedure. In the estimated worst case of E ~40 mSv the risk would increase by 0,2%. Although low, the risks of developing an early transient erythema or a cancer cannot to be totally disregarded. All attempts should therefore be made to control and minimise dose to the patient (see below).

Fluoroscopic guidance allows KP to be performed in the operating theatre with the advantage of optimal sterility and the option of operative intervention in the event of complications. Although data for comparison is lacking, it is unlikely that comparable fractures could be treated with lesser E-values through CT guided KP as repeated scanning and additional fluoroscopy during PMMA injection is usually necessary. It therefore appears justifiable to reserve CT guided KP for fractures with very poor visualisation, such as occasionally occur in the upper thoracic spine or in metastatic disease with extensive vertebral osteolysis.

Exposure is directed by the surgeon via foot pedals. As the entire finesse of the procedure is in the hands of the surgeon, this is the only way of optimising fluoroscopy exposure without endangering the patient and hampering the flow of the operation. It is highly doubtful, whether exposure guided by a radiology technician would have been able to achieve comparable values and would in any way have contributed positively to the success of the procedure.

A reduction of ET can be achieved through pulsed imaging. The concern of missing PMMA leakage however usually prompts surgeons to use non-pulsed imaging in short bursts. Nevertheless, pulsed imaging should be used where justifiable (e.g. for tool introduction). Studies will need to be directed towards comparing the risk of PMMA leakage in pulsed and non-pulsed imaging before formulating recommendations in this regard. Although employing adjustable diaphragms would reduce E, they are usually not used as the entire circumference of the vertebral body must remain well visualised during PMMA injection in order to detect any prevertebral venous leakage that could lead to pulmonary embolism. Further technical measures to reduce patient dose in KP include operating the fluoroscopes at the highest level of image intensifier sensitivity, which is acceptable for this intervention. The most suitable characteristic curve should be selected to govern the control mode of the automatic brightness control unit. With regard to patient dose, characteristic curves are preferable, which increase tube voltage to enhance the x-ray output, compensating for increased patient thickness. Use should be made of the lock-in switch once the automatic brightness control unit has established tube voltage and tube current according to patient thickness. This measure prevents readjustment of x-ray output towards higher values, when contrast media and tools enter the x-ray beam. C-arms with large spans should be used and the patient should be positioned as close to the image intensifier as practically possible. This mainly helps to reduce ESD. Finally, the fluoroscopes should be regularly inspected, to ensure their proper function and the operating team should be familiar with the control mode of the automatic brightness control unit and the consequences of this device for patient dose and image quality.

References

Boszczyk BM, Bierschneider M, Panzer S, Panzer W, Harstall R, Schmid K, Jaksche H (2006) Fluoroscopic radiation exposure of the kyphoplasty patient. Eur Spine J 15(3): 347–55

Harstall R, Heini PF, Mini RL, Orler R (2004) Radiation exposure to the surgeon during fluoroscopically assisted percutaneous vertebroplasty: a prospective study. Spine 30(16): 1893–8

Wagner LK, Eifel PJ, Geise RA (1994) Potential Biological Effects Following High X-ray Dose Interventional Procedures. J Vasc Interv Radiol 5: 71–84

Chapter 8

Results in kyphoplasty, risks and complications

U. Berlemann, P. Hulme, and O. Schwarzenbach

During recent years kyphoplasty has gained increasing importance in the treatment of osteoporotic vertebral body fractures. In addition to the pain-relieving effect, the possibility of reducing the fracture and thus preserving the spinal alignment is advantageous. Patients with these fractures often suffer from chronic pain, as well as the acute pain, because of the increasing kyphotic condition of the vertebral body and the resulting deviation of the spine. The change in spinal alignment correlates with restricted mobility and loss of quality of life, leading to the increased mortality rate following vertebral body fractures [Lyles 1993]. Furthermore, these parameters get progressively worse, with an increasing number of vertebrae affected and the resulting increase of the positional failure [Ross 1997]. It would be invaluable for those affected if this development could not only be stopped but even reversed with minimally invasive technology causing little stress to the patients. Kyphoplasty claims to already fulfil many features of such a technology. The impression given by individual articles on the clinical results of kyphoplasty is extremely positive, though because of the large number of recently published articles it is easy to lose track. The following questions arise:

- How do the published results look if they are brought together systematically?
- How must the results of kyphoplasty be judged in comparison with vertebroplasty?
- Does kyphoplasty really fulfil the requirement to durably improve the position of the sintered vertebral body?
- And if so, is there a measurable advantage for the patient?
- What problems and complications arise during the time following an initially successful kyphoplasty?
- In particular, how do adjacent segments and further vertebral bodies react?

This chapter will try to find answers to these questions on the basis of published data and will evaluate the current clinical standing of kyphoplasty.

Materials and methods

Published clinical data on kyphoplasty were systematically analyzed and relevant parameters were compared with data on vertebroplasty. The sources used were Medline, The Cochrane Library and Current Contents, in which articles containing the keywords "vertebroplasty" and "kyphoplasty" were searched as of November 1, 2004. A total of 530 articles were identified. After excluding biomechanical studies, review articles, editorials, articles in languages other than English, French, German or Spanish, 44 articles on vertebroplasty and 19 on kyphoplasty remained for further evaluation [Berlemann 2004; Coumans 2003; Crandall 2004; Darius 2003; Dudeney 2002; Fourney 2003; Fribourg 2004; Harrop 2004; Hillmeier 2004a, b; Kornp 2004; Lane 2004; Ledlie 2003; Lieberman 2001; Phillips 2003; Rhyne 2004; Theodorou 2002; Weisskopf 2003; Wilhelm 2003]. These were assessed by at least two reviewers using a modified version of the quality assessment tool of Downs and Black [Downs 1998]. This tool contains all the criteria for assessment of scientific work used by the leading institutions and agencies in this field; e.g. the Agency for Healthcare Research and Quality (AHRQ), the Cochrane Collaboration Back Review Group and the NHS R&D Health Technology Assessment Program. Various criteria were evaluated and individually awarded points; a maximum total score of 29 points was possible. The morphological data and results described in the articles were summarized and evaluated according to the following subpoints:

- Pain relief
- General health
- Improvements in function
- Satisfaction with treatment
- Repositioning of kyphosis
- Complications (especially cement extrusions)
- New fractures

Not every article dealt with each sub-point, therefore the number of cases that could be evaluated was reduced accordingly in some articles.

Results

The quality of the evaluated work differed very much. The average rating of the articles was 16.6 points out of a possible 29 (standard deviation 3.9, range 6.5–23.5). Eleven of the 19 kyphoplasty articles were prospective studies. None of the studies fulfilled the criteria for randomization and only a few included a control group. In total, the results of 887 patients in 1624 kyphoplasties are described in the 19 articles. The average age of the patients was 71 (mean range 63.5–76), 65% of the patients were women, and 60% of the kyphoplasties were in the thoracic-lumbar region TV11–LV2.

The cited comparison data were taken from evaluation of 44 articles on vertebroplasty. These dealt with the treatment of 4827 vertebral bodies in 3325 patients. The demographic data were similar to those for the kyphoplasty group.

Pain relief

The proportion of patients who experienced pain relief after kyphoplasty was very high at 91% (95% confidence interval (CI) 93–99%), slightly higher than after vertebroplasty (86%, 77–95%). Pain relief was typically experienced very early, either immediately after the operation or within a few days. The VAS decreased from 7.25 (95% CI ± 0.55) to 3.2 (95% CI ± 0.69), roughly corresponding with the results for vertebroplasty. Only three studies also reported SF-36 scores; in these the value for pain dropped by 22.4 points to 47.1 and the value for function dropped by 17.2 points to 29.3. No differences could be shown in the areas of general or mental health.

Correction of kyphosis

The measurement and description of kyphosis correction is very inhomogeneous. Some studies measure the absolute height of the treated vertebral body, some express the height in relation to height before treatment or in relation to the adjacent vertebra. The percentage improvement varies from 12.9% to 47%. The degree of the kyphosis correction is also described very inhomogeneously, adding to the wide range of results which vary from 15.1% to 50.2%. Table 7 shows the results of the individual articles. A good third of the treatments did not show any visible repositioning of the vertebra, i.e. the alteration was less than 5° and thus lay within the area of the measuring error. Varying results are described for the loss of the repositioning: in some cases practically no recurrence of kyphosis is described, whereas Hillmeier describes losses of up to 44% of the initial gain in height [Hillmeier 2004b].

Almost no details are given on the success of repositioning in vertebroplasty. Some of the articles describe a subgroup of "mobile fractures" that achieve similar repositioning results to kyphoplasty by positioning the patient properly [Jang 2003; Lee 2004; McKiernan 2003]. The rate of the "failures," i.e. the cases without certain repositioning (< 5°), is also of interest and varied from 22.2% to 89% of kyphoplasty cases, with a corresponding rate of 28.5% to 64.6% for vertebroplasty.

Complications

The rate of clinically relevant complications reached 1% of the treated vertebral bodies in kyphoplasty and 2.7% in vertebroplasty. However, problems in placing the instruments must be distinguished from problems of cement extrusion from the vertebral body. The rate of extrusions was 8.5% (CI 1.6–15.3%) for kyphoplasty but 36.8% for vertebroplasty (CI 27.7–46%). Nevertheless, most of these extrusions were clinically asymptomatic and the rate of serious problems remains low, e.g. the risk of pulmonary embolism is 0.01% in kyphoplasty and 0.6% in vertebroplasty.

New fractures

Nine clinical studies on kyphoplasty and 13 on vertebroplasty gave information on the occurrence of new fractures. However, because of varying course durations, exact calculation of the rate per time unit was practically impossible and therefore any significant difference between the two techniques could not be seen from the data. Nevertheless, it can be stated that 60–67% of the new fractures occurred directly next to an augmented vertebra and that

Results in kyphoplasty, risks and complications

Table 7. Balloon kyphoplasty – reduction of the vertebral body height and kyphosis

Study	Duration of symptoms (months)	Number of vertebral bodies	Patients with no change of kyphosis (%)	Middle range improved (%) [method‡]	Reduction of kyphosis		
					Correction (%)	Pre-Op angle (degree)	Post-Op angle (degree)
Berlemann et al. 2004	1 (2–180 days)	27 (mobil)	22.2	–	47.7	17 ± 6.6	9 ± 5
Crandall et al. 2004	< 10 weeks > 4 months	40 46 (MRI)	8 20	28 [4] 23 [4]	47 33	15 15	8 10
Darius et al. 2003	–	8	–	–	34	–	–
Dudeney et al. 2002	11 (0.5–24)	39 (MRI)	31	34 [3]	–	–	–
Fourney et al. 2003	3.2† (0.25–26)	37 (MRI)	–	42 ± 21 [3]	16	25.7 ± 9.7	20 ± 8.7
Hillmeier et al. 2004a	all (a) < 4 wk (b) > 4 wk	173 (a) 20 (b) 153	50 (0–10%)	Mean = 10.3 (a) 20 [4] (b) 9 [4]	–	–	–
Hillmeier et al. 2004b	(a) < 4 wk (b) > 4 wk	192 (a) 20 (b) 172	–	Mean = 10 (a) 18 [4] (b) 9 [4]2	–	–	–
Lane et al. 2004	> 3 (90%)	46 (meta) 37 (osteo)	9 0	53.4 ± 29* [3] 60.3 ± 29 [3]			
Ledie and Renfro 2003	2.4 (0–14)	26 (acute frakt.)	–	25 [4]	–	–	–
Lieberman et al. 2001	5.9 (0.5–24)	70 (MRI)	30 (height)	35 [3] 46.8* [3]	–	–	–
Phillips et al. 2003	3.8 (0.9–12.3)	52 (oedema)	42.3	–	50.2	17.5	8.7
Rhyne III et al.	1 (0.2–27.7)	82 2004 (oedema MRI)	–	23.2 [2]	15.1	22.5	19.1
Theodorou et al. 2002	3.27 (0.5–11)	24 (acute)	–	26.1 [2]§ 65.7 ± 36 [3] 12.9 [4]	38.8§	25.5 ± 10	15.6 ± 6.7
Weisskopf et al. 2003	–	37	89	–	–	–	–
Wilhelm et al. 2003	2.26 (0.4–72)	56	–	–	56.5	11.5	5

All values represented as mean ± SD. "No change of kyphyosis" is defined as changes less than 5° between the pre- and post-operative angles. ‡ % height restoration, method according to McKiernan et al., 2003. Method 1: Absolute height restoration in mm. Method 2: Proportional height restoration relative to the initial fracture height. Method 3: Proportional height restoration relative to the height loss of the vertebral body. Method 4: Proportional height restoration relative to another vertebral body as reference. Method 5: Proportional height in relation to the height of a reference vertebral body. § Calculated from the available data. *Data concerning those vertebral bodies for which a repositioning of the vertebral body height could be detected.

most new fractures were seen within the first six months after the intervention.

Discussion

This overview encompassed 19 studies that included a total of 887 patients who underwent 1624 kyphoplasties overall. In addition, the data were compared with those for vertebroplasty, with records on 3325 patients and 4827 treated levels. The most striking point when analyzing the studies was the great lack of homogeneity in aspects such as patient recruitment, methodical procedure, and evaluation and presentation of results. This not only has a negative effect on the validity of the publications but makes comparisons much more difficult. Nonetheless, it was possible to draw up a catalog according to which future treatments should be documented and evaluated:

– Preoperative MRI to determine the activity of the injury, at least in cases with unclear age of the fracture;
– Preoperative functional image in order to determine the mobility of the fracture;
– Postoperative thorough analysis of cement extrusions, possibly by means of CT;
– Postoperative assessment of kyphosis reduction by means of measurement of height of both the treated vertebral body and its intact neighbor, as well as measurement of the angle of the treated vertebral body and the appropriate segment of the spine (including the cranial intervertebral disc);
– Radiological examination to identify new fractures after 6 weeks, 3 months and 6 months;
– Clinical documentation by means of VAS, SF36 and Oswestry scores, preoperatively and then after 6 weeks, 3 months, 6 months and 12 months.

A further important point is that not a single prospective randomized study has yet been published that compares kyphoplasty directly with vertebroplasty, nor either technique with conservative treatment.

Despite these restrictions some aspects can be clearly derived from the studies analyzed in this review.

Both kyphoplasty and vertebroplasty are very successful pain-relieving methods. This applies at least for the short-term course (< 1 year). The mechanism of pain reduction is most likely to lie in the mechanical stabilization of the fractured vertebral body, as there are no essential differences between the curing properties of the various cements. Until now, details on the question of when to expect complete pain relief, as opposed to those few cases where patients show no pain reduction at all, could not be determined. Follow-up observations of more than a year are still scarce; however, there are no indications that a positive result showing after one year changes essentially later on [Zoarski 2002].

There is only one non-randomized prospective study that has compared vertebroplasty with conservative treatment [Diamond 2003]. Directly after treatment of acute fractures the vertebroplasty patients had considerably less pain, but after only six weeks the results for the two groups were similar again.

Direct comparison of kyphoplasty and vertebroplasty is also rare. In a more recently published paper, which was not included in the present analysis, the two techniques gave similar pain-relieving results but more cement extrusions were observed with vertebroplasty (DeNegri 2007).

This advantage of kyphoplasty could also be clearly shown in the analysis: the risk of cement extrusion was considerably higher with vertebroplasty, by a factor of 4–5. In kyphoplasty relatively viscous cement can be used, which allows controlled filling of a cavity in the vertebral body, and this considerably reduces the risk of cement leakage. This is an advantage not only with respect to potentially immediately dangerous extrusions into the spinal canal or to embolism but also for initially clinically asymptomatic cement leakages that may have negative long-term effects. A considerably higher rate of fractures of adjacent segments could be established in cases of intradiscal cement extrusions [Lin 2004].

Fractures of further vertebral bodies represent the largest clinical problem in the treatment after augmentation with cement, and certainly also determine the long-term outcome. Adequate treatment of osteoporosis as the basic disease is of crucial importance in the interdisciplinary approach. However, in individual cases the question will always arise of whether a new fracture is due to the natural course of the condition or whether it has been provoked biomechanically by the augmented vertebral body. Whether there are any differences between vertebroplasty and kyphoplasty in this risk cannot be determined from the available data. Reduction of kyphosis of the affected segment combined with relief of the anterior column should at least theoretically reduce the risk of subsequent fractures. The consequences of the distribution of the cement, either diffusely within the vertebral body (vertebroplasty) or as a bolus (kyphoplasty), on biomechanical reactions have yet to be examined more closely.

Reports on the success of repositioning with these augmentation methods vary considerably. The age of the fracture has been highlighted as an important criterion for kyphoplasty [Berlemann 2004; Lieberman 2001], in the sense that old or already osseous strongly consolidated fractures can no longer be reduced. On the other hand, repositioning of fractures not older than 6–8 weeks is usually quite successful (Table 7). The possibility of height restoration of the vertebral body is also described for vertebroplasty, and in cases of "mobile fractures" achieves results that are quite comparable to those of kyphoplasty. However, this is achieved through postural mechanisms of the patient on the operating table, as the technique of vertebroplasty, unlike kyphoplasty, does not offer any intrinsic possibility of fracture repositioning. The actual benefit of the direct internal raising of the vertebral body with balloons has been examined only recently and has shown that the use of a kyphoplasty balloon tamp is superior to postural correction alone (Shindle 2006).

The question of loss of repositioning in the further course has also been evaluated in different ways. Some articles describe no essential loss after kyphoplasty [Berlemann 2004; Ledlie 2003], whereas others report sintering, at least in individual cases of acute fractures [Hillmeier 2004b].

Details on how the application of cement effects the overall alignment of the spine are also missing from recent studies. In future it would be desirable to take this into account by taking survey radiographs of the spine, as the overall posture of the spine is of greater significance for the patient than the condition of a single segment [Lieberman 2001].

At present, the questions asked at the beginning of the chapter can be answered as follows:

Kyphoplasty is a very successful method for reduction of pain in osteoporotic vertebral body fractures, and in that respect is not greatly different from vertebroplasty. In addition, the complication rate in kyphoplasty, especially regarding the risk of cement extrusion, is significantly lower than in vertebroplasty.

Improvements in the positioning of the vertebral body can be achieved in two-thirds of all kyphoplasty cases. In certain cases of "mobile fractures" the improvement partially occurs through appropriate positioning of the patient, which similarly leads to height restoration in the appropriate subgroup of vertebroplasty cases.

Proof that this repositioning is advantageous to the patient, compared with applying cement "in situ," has yet to be confirmed.

The biggest clinical problem in the follow-up after kyphoplasty is the occurrence of new fractures; however, in this respect it is still unclear whether there are any differences between the two techniques.

It is interesting to note that further recently published reviews reach conclusions similar to those of the present data analysis [Taylor 2006, 2007].

References

Alanay A (2003) Early radiographic and clinical results of balloon kyphoplasty for the treatment of osteoporotic vertebral compression fractures – Point of view. Spine 28: 2265–7

Berlemann U, Franz T, Orler R, Heini PF (2004) Kyphoplasty for treatment of osteoporotic vertebral fractures: a prospective non-randomized study. Eur Spine J 13: 496–501

Coumans JV, Reinhardt MK, Lieberman IH (2003) Kyphoplasty for vertebral compression fractures: 1-year clinical outcomes from a prospective study. J Neurosurg 99(15): 44–50

Crandall D, Slaughter D, Hankins PJ, Moore C, Jerman J (2004) Acute versus chronic vertebral compression fractures treated with kyphoplasty: early results. Spine J 4: 418–24

Darius T, Vanderschot P, Broos P (2003) Balloonkyfoplastiek: Een Nieuwe Behandelingsmethode voor Wevelfracturen bij Osteoporose. Tijdschr voor Geneeskunde 59, 19: 1141–51

De Negri P, Tirri T, Paternoster G, Modano P (2007) Treatment of painful osteoporotic or traumatic vertebral compression fractures by percutaneous vertebral augmentation procedures: a nonrandomized comparison between vertebroplasty and kyphoplasty. Clin J Pain 23(5): 425–30

Diamond TH, Champion B, Clark WA (2003) Management of acute osteoporotic vertebral fractures: a nonrandomized trial comparing percutaneous vertebroplasty with conservative therapy. Am J Med 114: 257–65

Downs SH, Black N (1998) The feasibility of creating a checklist for the assessment of the methodological quality both of randomised and non-randomised studies of health care interventions. J Epidemiol Community Health 52: 377–84

Dudeney S, Lieberman IH, Reinhardt MK, Hussein M (2002) Kyphoplasty in the treatment of osteolytic vertebral compression fractures as a result of multiple myeloma. J Clin Oncol 20: 2382–7

Fourney DR, Schomer DF, Nader R, et al (2003) Percutaneous vertebroplasty and kyphoplasty for painful vertebral body fractures in cancer patients. J Neurosurg 98: 21–30

Fribourg D, Tang C, Sra P, Delamarter R, Bae H (2004) Incidence of subsequent vertebral fracture after kyphoplasty. Spine 29: 2270–6

Harrop JS, Prpa B, Reinhardt MK, Lieberman I (2004) Primary and secondary osteoporosis' incidence of subsequent vertebral compression fractures after kyphoplasty. Spine 29: 2120–5

Hillmeier J, Grafe I, Da Fonseca K, et al (2004) Die Wertigkeit der Ballonkyphoplastie bei der osteoporotischen Wirbelkörperfraktur: ein interdisziplinäres Konzept. Orthopäde 33: 893–904

Hillmeier J, Meeder PJ, Noldge G, Kock HJ, Da Fonseca K, Kasperk HC (2004) Augmentation von Wirbelkörperfrakturen mit einem neuen Calciumphosphat-Zement nach Ballon-Kyphoplastie. Orthopäde 33: 31–9

Jang JS, Kim DY, Lee SH (2003) Efficacy of percutaneous vertebroplasty in the treatment of intravertebral pseudarthrosis associated with noninfected avascular necrosis of the vertebral body. Spine 28: 1588–92

Kornp M, Ruetten S, Godolias G (2004) Minimal-invasive Therapie der funktionell instabilen osteoporotischen Wirbelkörperfraktur mittels Kyphoplastie: Prospektive Vergleichsstudie von 19 operierten und 17 konservative behandelten Patienten. J Miner Stoffwechs 11/1: 13–5

Lane JM, Hong R, Koob J, et al (2004) Kyphoplasty enhances function and structural alignment in multiple myeloma. Clin Orthop 426: 49–53

Ledlie JT, Renfro M (2003) Balloon kyphoplasty: one-year outcomes in vertebral body height restoration, chronic pain, and activity levels. J Neurosurg 99: 36–42

Lee ST, Chen JF (2004) Closed reduction vertebroplasty for the treatment of osteoporotic vertebral compression fractures. Technical note. J Neurosurg 100: 392–6

Lieberman IH, Dudeney S, Reinhardt MK, Bell G (2001) Initial outcome and efficacy of "kyphoplasty" in the treatment of painful osteoporotic vertebral compression fractures. Spine 26: 1631–8

Lin EP, Ekholm S, Hiwatashi A, Westesson PL (2004) Vertebroplasty: cement leakage into the disc increases the risk of new fracture of adjacent vertebral body. AJNR Am J Neuroradiol 25: 175–80

Lyles KW, Gold DT, Shipp KM, Pieper CF, Martinez S, Mulhausen PL (1993) Association of osteoporotic vertebral compression fractures with impaired functional status. Am J Med 94: 595–601

McKiernan F, Faciszewski T, Jensen R (2003) Reporting height restoration in vertebral compression fractures. Spine 28: 2517–21

Phillips FM, Ho E, Campbell-Hupp M, McNally T, Todd WF, Gupta P (2003) Early radiographic and clinical results of balloon kyphoplasty for the treatment of osteoporotic vertebral compression fractures. Spine 28: 2260–5

Rhyne A, III, Banit D, Laxer E, Odum S, Nussman D (2004) Kyphoplasty: report of eighty-two thoracolumbar osteoporotic vertebral fractures. J Orthop Trauma 18: 294–9

Ross PD (1997) Clinical consequence of vertebral fractures. Am J Med 98: 30S–42S

Shindle MK, Gardner MJ, Koob J, Bukata S, Cabin JA, Lane JM (2006) Vertebral height restoration in osteoporotic compression fractures: kyphoplasty balloon tamp is superior to postural correction alone. Osteoporos Int 17(12): 1815–9

Taylor RS, Taylor RJ, Fritzell P (2006) Balloon kyphoplasty and vertebroplasty for vertebral compression fractures: a comparative systematic review of efficacy and safety. Spine 31(23): 2747–55

Taylor RS, Fritzell P, Taylor RJ (2007) Balloon kyphoplasty in the management of vertebral compression fractures: an updated systematic review and meta-analysis. Eur Spine J (in print)

Theodorou DJ, Theodorou SJ, Duncan TD, Garfin SR, Wong WH (2002) Percutaneous balloon kyphoplasty for the correction of spinal deformity in painful vertebral body compression fractures. Clin Imaging 26: 1–5

Weisskopf M, Herlein S, Birnbaum K, Siebert C, Stanzel S, Wirtz DC (2003) Kyphoplastie – ein neues minimalinvasives Verfahren zur Aufrichtung und Stabilisierung von Wirbelkörpern. Z Orthop Ihre Grenzgeb 142: 406–11

Wilhelm K, Stoffel M, Ringel F, et al (2003) Ballon-Kyphoplastie zur Behandlung schmerzhafter osteoporotischer Wirbelkörperfrakturen – Technik und erste Ergebnisse. Rofo Fortschr Geb Rontgenstr N 175: 1690–6

Zoarski GH, Snow P, Olan WJ, et al (2002) Percutaneous vertebroplasty for osteoporotic compression fractures: quantitative prospective evaluation of long-term outcomes. J Vasc Interv Radiol 13: 139–48

Summary: the risks of kyphoplasty

M. Bierschneider, B. Boszczyk, and H. Jaksche

The risks of kyphoplasty and the procedure presented here also apply to vertebroplasty, a simpler technique with direct uni- or bipedicular injection of cement into the vertebral body without the introduction of a balloon. The techniques of vertebroplasty and lordoplasty, a minimally invasive further development, are explained below in chapter 11.

In principle, both kyphoplasty and vertebroplasty carry possible risks at all levels of decision and action, i.e. pre-, intra- and postoperatively.

1. Preoperative risks

If a minimally invasive augmentation method is indicated, the therapist should ask the following questions:

- The right method?
- The right patient?
- The right surgeon?
- The right vertebra?
- The right material?

1.1 The right method?

Neither vertebroplasty nor kyphoplasty are suited in principle to replace the established methods of spinal surgery for traumatic fractures. However, they can represent an alternative to conservative treatment as well as to open surgery for selected patients. The indication for vertebro- or kyphoplasty is restricted to patients with fractures of types A 1.1 and A 1.2 and to selected cases of type A 3.1. Great caution is advised in all cases of spinal or foraminal stenosis accompanied by any clinical loss of function (spinal claudication, radicular failures), as cement injection cannot help with these problems.

1.2 The right patient?

A minimally invasive method does not turn an inoperable patient into an operable one.

The patient must be capable of receiving a general anesthetic or, if the operation is to be carried out under local anesthesia, at least be able to lie in an abdominal position for the duration of the operation. In cases of severe adiposis, the identification of anatomical marks necessary for placing the instruments and the observation of the bone cement during injection could be so difficult that it is not safe to carry out this procedure. This particularly applies to the high thoracic region and the lumbosacral area because adjacent anatomical structures (shoulders, pelvis) make radiological superposition possible.

Furthermore, the following absolute contraindications must be observed for both methods when selecting patients:

1. Asymptomatic vertebral body fractures;
2. Treatment-refractory coagulopathy or hemorrhagic diathesis;
3. Bacterial infections.

1.3 The right surgeon?

The surgeon should have sufficient experience in operating the spine and should have participated in a theoretical-practical course for learning the technique of vertebro- or kyphoplasty. In addition the surgeon should be capable of treating complications that require switching to open surgery.

1.4 The right vertebra?

Great care must be taken to identify the correct vertebra responsible for the pain. This is frequently difficult in elderly patients as they often have a long-standing case history with backache and thus corresponding degenerative changes appear on the initial x-ray.

The x-ray, the sector-scan and the clinical pain of the patient must correlate.

In clinical practice, magnetic resonance imaging has proven to be extremely helpful in identification of bone edema in the vertebral body in cases of doubt. A variety of bone cement is available. In order to be suitable for vertebro- or kyphoplasty the material must fulfil defined requirements: it must have good injecting qualities, adequate radiological visualization, a time frame of approx. 10–12 minutes for processing, and provide sufficient primary stability. Cements primarily used are based on polymethylmethacrylate. Comparable results have also been achieved with calcium phosphate cements for osteoporotic fractures. The suitability of calcium phosphate cements for traumatic fractures in young people is currently being investigated.

2. Intraoperative risks

Two types of intraoperative risk can be primarily distinguished: risks caused by the access and risks caused by applying cement.

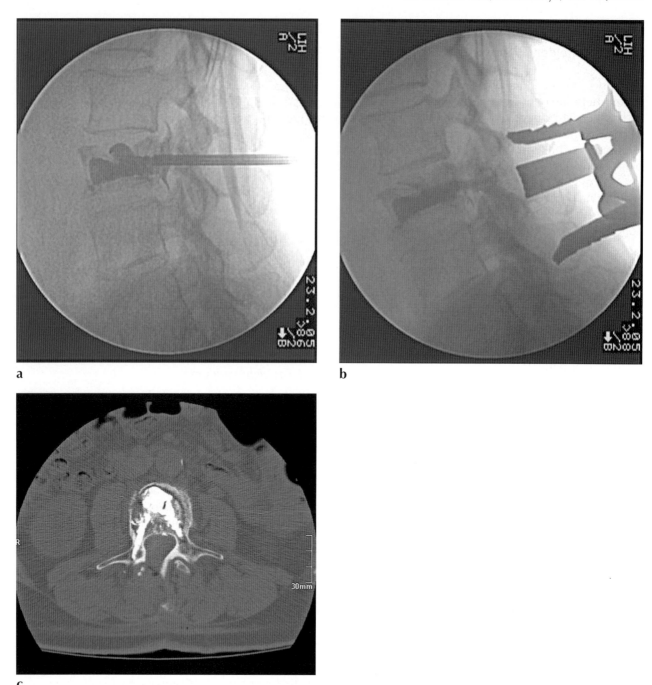

Fig. 43. A 59-year-old patient, in pain since 10/2004, CT of lumbar spine 2/2005: Fracture L3. Percutaneous bilateral balloon kyphoplasty of L3 on February 23, 2005. During the operation one balloon protruded into the intervertebral space, so the expansion was stopped and the balloon on the opposite side kept in place while filling the cement. After filling the cavern on the opposite side, the balloon was deflated and removed. While filling the balloon on the right hand side, cement leaked into the spinal canal (**a**). The amount of cement that had leaked seemed to be too much to be left unattended, therefore the spinal canal was opened via an extended fenestration and the cement removed (**b**). The cement was located on the medial pedicle wall and could be removed effortlessly with the rongeur (**c**). A big epidural vein had caused the leakage. The patient had no postoperative neurological deficits even though the cement had already hardened at the time it was removed

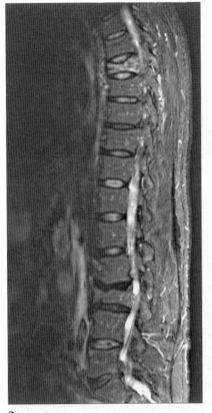
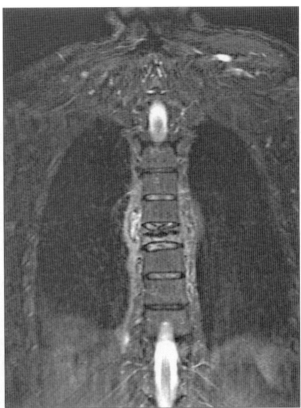
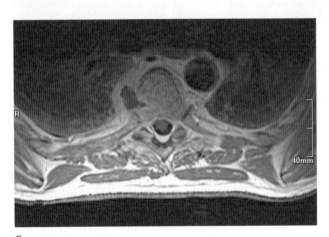

Fig. 44. A 47-year-old man, who fell during a game of curling on March 4, 2004. The MRI shows acute fracture of T7. He underwent percutaneous unilateral balloon kyphoplasty on March 18, 2004 and was discharged painless on March 22, 2004. After 2 days of increasing thoracic pain, he presented in the outpatient department on March 30, 2004. The MRI shows a perivertebral inflammation reaction with abscess of T6/7 (**a–c**). He was treated with antibiotics, hyperbaric oxygen and a corset. Slow recovery from pain in the course of a year, but increase of the malposition and pain when stress on the anterior column. The patient was offered a ventro-dorsal stabilization which he declined

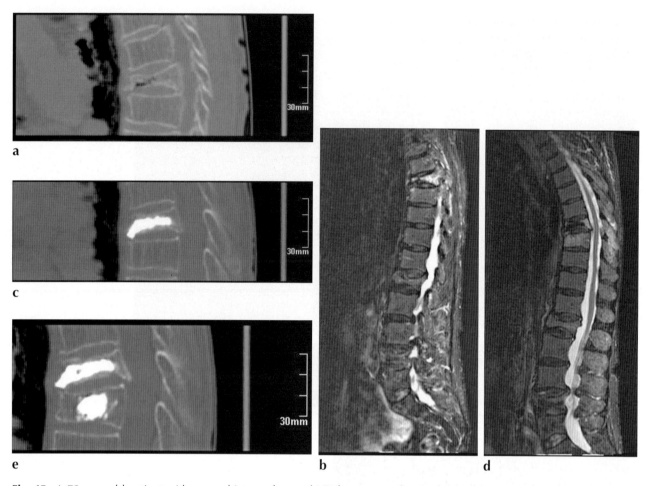

Fig. 45. A 78-year-old patient with a case history of several VB fractures and acute backache since 3 days ago. The preoperative MRI shows acute fracture of T8 (**a**, **b**). Percutaneous unilateral balloon kyphoplasty performed from the right (**c**). During mobilization, renewed postoperative pain immediately in the area of the operation entrance. Control MRI shows a subsequent fracture of T9 (**d**). Percutaneous unilateral balloon kyphoplasty of T9 performed from the right (**e**), distinct postoperative recovery from pain

In principle all structures and organs within and surrounding the spine are in danger of being injured while the cannula is pushed forward, under x-ray guidance, into the appropriate vertebral body. Medial deviation of the cannula can perforate the spinal canal and injure the spinal cord or the cauda equina, with corresponding neurological failures. Lateral deviation of the cannula could possibily perforate the lungs or the abdominal organs, depending which segment of the spine is being treated. An anterior perforation could possibly lead to injury of the big vessels.

Nevertheless, the injury rate for structures surrounding the route into the vertebral body is considerably under 1% for both methods, although the number of unrecorded cases carried out by less experienced practitioners seems to lie considerably higher.

Bad imaging and insufficient experience of the surgeon are considered the main causes of injury to adjacent structures.

Cement leakage is the most frequent complication in both methods (Fig. 43). Cement can leak into the spinal canal, the neuroforamina, the surrounding muscular system, as well as into the blood vessels and then spread into the lungs. The leakage rate varies considerably between the two methods: from 10–70% for vertebroplasty, to less than 10% for kyphoplasty. The much higher rate of cement leakage in vertebroplasty is due to the difference in the technology.

In vertebroplasty thin cement is injected into the trabeculate bone under a high pressure; in kyphoplasty viscous cement is brought under low pressure into a cavity created by a balloon. The reasons for cement leakage can be, apart from too thin a cement and too high an injection pressure, bad imaging during the injection phase and impatience on the part of the surgeon during the injection.

In order to avoid cement leakage it is therefore recommended that the cement is injected as viscous as possible, without force, without haste, and with good imaging.

3. Postoperative risks

The postoperative risks are primarily infections and a subsequent fracture.

3.1 Infection (Fig. 44)

Postoperative infection can appear locally as wound infection in the access area, or it can extend into the paravertebral soft tissue, break into the spinal canal, or involve the vertebral bodies or the intervertebral disc.

There are various factors that predispose a patient to postoperative infection. Immunosuppression, diabetes mellitus and adiposis have to be mentioned first, but sterility failures during preparation and performance of the operation must also be taken into account.

In order to minimize the risk of infection, patients should be selected according to their personal risk profile, taking contraindications into consideration and using paraoperative antibiotic prophylaxis if necessary. The operation should of course be performed in an adequately equipped operating room, and with the usual hygienic precautions for operations.

3.2 Connecting fracture (Fig. 45)

Of new fractures that occur, 30–60% are adjacent. There is an increased risk of connecting fractures in cases of multiple pre-existing fractures and in secondary osteoporosis. As far as we know today this can be interpreted as follows:

The risk of a connecting fracture is determined by the extent of the basic osteoporotic condition.

Consistent treatment of the basic disease improves matters here.

Conclusion

Minimally invasive technology does not mean minimal risk.

The risks can be calculated if the operation is performed by an experienced surgeon who has access to good imaging in an adequately equipped operating room with the possibility of treating complications.

We see the main risk as the uncritical expansion of the indications by surgeons who do not have sufficient experience in operating the spine.

Chapter 9

Special indications and techniques of balloon kyphoplasty

S. Becker and M. Ogon

In this chapter we describe special techniques that are required in difficult situations. The normal balloon kyphoplasty technique has to be modified in cases of neurological deficits with compression of the spinal cord or nerve roots and in the case of metastatic changes. Of course it is up to the surgeon to combine the conventional balloon kyphoplasty technique with an open reduction in the case of compression syndromes (Fig. 48) in order to avoid an anterior operation.

Balloon kyphoplasty for the treatment of malignant bone tumors

In principle primary and secondary bone tumors have to be distinguished.

Plasmocytoma (multiple myeloma)

Multiply myeloma represents 50% of all primary tumors of the spine. This type of tumor also plays the most important role among our own balloon kyphoplasty patients. Multiple myeloma causes bone resorption by stimulating the osteoclasts via the osteoclast activating factor [Callander 2001]. This usually leads to a diffuse condition of the spine with painful progressive vertebral compression fractures at several levels [Dudeney 2002]. However, in the last few years the survival rate of multiple myeloma patients has increased significantly as a result of further development and improvement in chemotherapy [Barlogie 1999; Berenson 1996]. In particular, bone morbidity is significantly lowered by simultaneously administering bisphosphonates [Berenson 1996]. Patients with multiple myeloma are thus ideal candidates for balloon kyphoplasty and first experiences have proved very satisfactory [Dudeney 2002]; significant postoperative improvement in the SF-36 score (life quality questionnaire [McHorney 1993; Ware 1992]) has been achieved.

Regarding the prophylactic use of balloon kyphoplasty in multiple myeloma patients without vertebral fracture, it is difficult to assess whether or not they will suffer a fracture in the future. No prophylactic kyphoplasties have been performed in these patients but it is imaginable that, in cases where chemotherapy fails, early direct stabilization of the spine could be carried out.

Osteolytic metastases

The spine is the part of the skeleton that is most frequently affected by metastases. In particular, osteolytic metastasis with a spontaneous fracture can be misinterpreted as an osteoporotic vertebral body fracture. We therefore take a biopsy with the bone-filler or with the biopsy trocar in every balloon kyphoplasty before inserting the balloon (Chapter 7, Fig. 21).

Of all cases of the spine affected by metastases, only osteolytic metastases are suitable for balloon kyphoplasty. In the case of osteoblastic metastasis there is a risk that the metastases are pushed into the spinal canal by the balloon. Furthermore, even though osteoblastic metastases are painful, they only seldom cause vertebral fractures, therefore the situation of the spine is primarily more stable. Osteolytic metastases, however, greatly endanger the stability of the spine and furthermore are very painful so that early operative intervention is required. Osteolytic metastases can be caused by primary carcinomata of the prostate, breast, stomach, lungs, kidneys and thyroid gland [Grundmann 1986]. The positive effect of the cement on osteolysis of vertebral bodies in adenocarcinoma of the lung and in multiple eosinophilic granuloma has already been described after vertebroplasty [Baba 1997; Cardon 1994]. First postoperative results after balloon kyphoplasty show significant pain relief lasting up to one year after the operation [Fourney 2003].

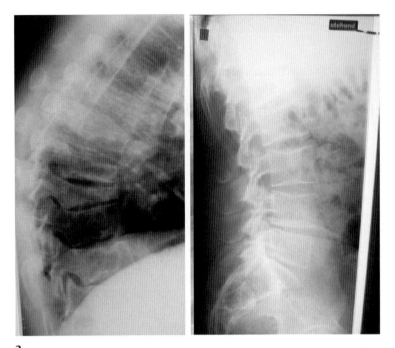

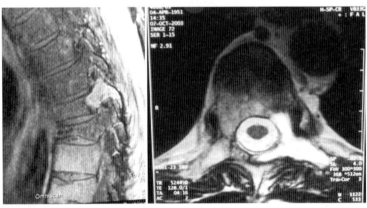

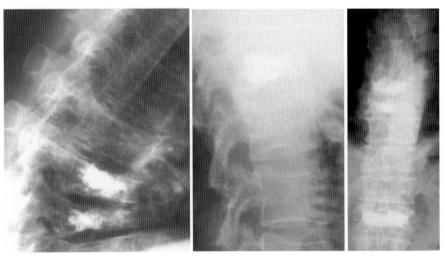

Fig. 46. A 53-year-old male, known plasmocytoma, condition after chemo- and radiotherapy with lesion of vertebrae T8, T9 and L1 (**a**), lesion of arch T8 (**b**), extrapedicular balloon kyphoplasty T8 and T9, transpedicular balloon kyphoplasty L1 (**c**)

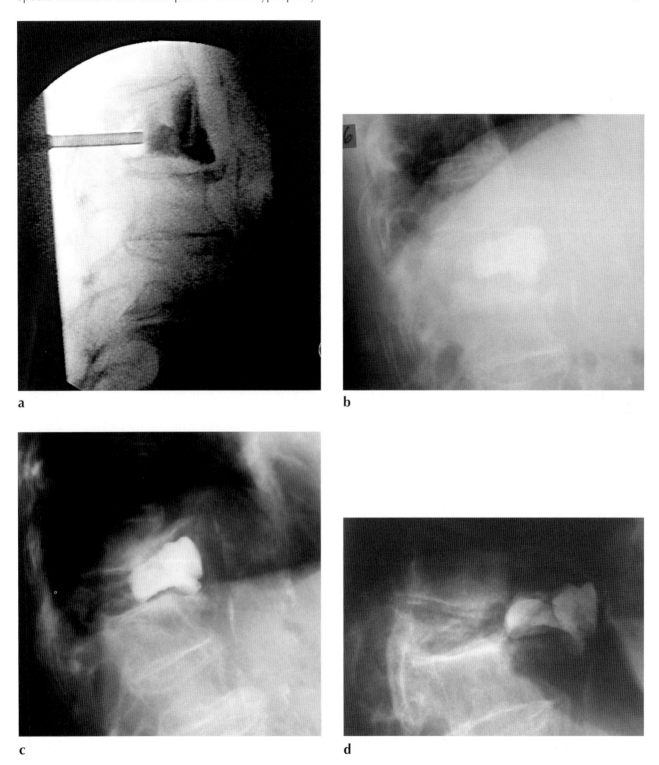

Fig. 47. An 83-year-old female, condition after vertebroplasty of T12 with osteolysis and unknown primary tumor. **a** Intraoperative picture. **b** Ventral dislocation of the cement beginning after 3 weeks. **c** Picture 9 months postoperative. **d** Results 2 years postoperative

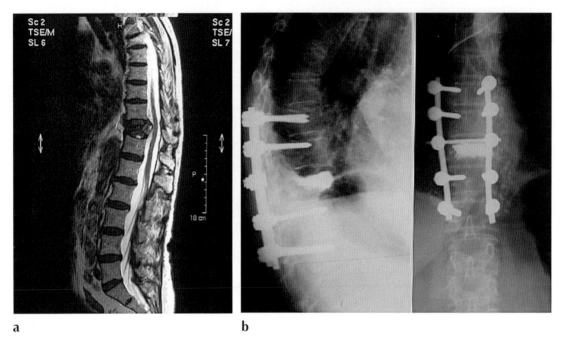

Fig. 48. a Female, metastatic vertebral body compression of T11 with unknown primary tumor, incomplete neurological failures of the lower extremities. Clear spinal stenosis. **b** Surgical treatment with laminectomy and open balloon kyphoplasty of T11 and dorsal instrumentation of T9 to L1 with dorsolateral cancellous bone graft

Another good indication for balloon kyphoplasty is a fracture caused by a hemangioma, a benign but painful lesion. Thus far, hemorrhagic problems have not been reported after stabilization of these lesions [Berlemann 2004; Castel 1999; Galibert 1990].

Special techniques in cases of plasmocytoma (multiple myeloma) and osteolytic metastases

Unlike vertebroplasty, balloon kyphoplasty is able to rebuild an osteolytic vertebral body wall by means of the egg-shell technique, which is described below. Nonetheless, in our experience it is more difficult to carry out balloon kyphoplasty in cases of vertebral metastases and plasmocytoma than it is in primary osteoporotic fractures. The risk of cement leakage is greater than in osteoporotic fractures, therefore the egg-shell technique (see below) should be preferred to the conventional balloon kyphoplasty technique (Fig. 54). Furthermore, there is the possibility that the pedicles are also affected by osteolysis, making transpedicular access no longer safe. In this case either a contralateral single approach via a still intact pedicle or an extrapedicular approach can be chosen (Fig. 46). The increased convergence of the balloon in the extrapedicular approach allows it to be placed centrally in the vertebra and a single balloon may be sufficient for the stabilization. Nevertheless, the possibility of dislocation of the cement block has to be taken into account if the anterior cortical substance is missing (Fig. 47).

In summary, balloon kyphoplasty combined with optimal oncologic therapy offers good possibility for stabilization of the osteolytic spine, especially in cases of plasmocytoma that have a good survival prognosis. Just as for patients with osteoporosis, quality of life and reduction of pain are the main objectives in treatment for tumor patients. Metastases on every level of the spine can be treated, and individual cases of cervical spine stabilization with cement have been reported [Wetzel 2002]. Furthermore, a combined method (Fig. 48) can also lead to a primary stable situation in metastatic conditions with neurological deficits; balloon kyphoplasty can be combined with a purely dorsal instrumentation and decompression thus avoiding a secondary anterior approach.

References

Baba Y, Ohkubo K, Hamada K, et al (1997) Percutaneous vertebroplasty for osteolytic metastasis: a case report. Nippon Igaku Hoshasen Gakkai Zasshi 57: 880–2

Barlogie B, Jagannath S, Desikan K, et al (1999) Total therapy with tandem transplants of newly diagnosed multiple myeloma. Blood 93: 55–5

Berenson A, Lichtenstein A, Porter L, et al (1996) Efficacy of palmidronate in reducing skeletal events in patients with advanced multiple myeloma. N Engl J Med 22; 334(8): 488–93

Berlemann U, Müller CW, Krettek C (2004) Perkutane Augmentierungtechniken der Wirbelsäule. Orthopäde 33(1): 6–12

Callander NS, Roodman GD (2001) Myeloma bone disease. Semin Hematol 38: 276–85

Cardon T, Hachulla E, Flipo RM, et al (1994) Percutaneous vertebroplasty with acrylic cement in the treatment of a Langerhans cell vertebral histiocytosis. Clin Rheumatol 13: 518–21

Castel E, Lazennec JY, Chiras J, et al (1999) Acute spinal cord compression due to intraspinal bleeding from a vertebral hemangioma: two case-reports. Eur Spine J 8: 244–48

Dudeney S, Lieberman IH, Reinhardt MK, Hussein M (2002) Kyphoplasty in the treatment of osteolytic vertebral compression fractures as a result of multiple myeloma. J Clin Oncol 20(9): 2382–7

Fourney DR, Schomer DF, Nader R, et al (2003) Percutaneous vertebroplasty and kyphoplasty for painful vertebral body fractures in cancer patients. J Neurosurg Spine 98(1): 21–30

Galibert P, Deramond H (1990) Percutaneos acrylic vertebroplasty as a treatment of vertebral angioma as well as painful and debilitating diseases. Chirurgie 116: 326–34

Grundmann E (1986) Spezielle Pathologie. Urban & Schwarzenberg, München

McHorney CA, Ware JE Jr, Raczek AE (1993) The MOS 36-Item Short-Form Health Survey (SF-36). II. Psychometric and clinical tests of validity in measuring physical and mental health constructs. Med Care 31(3): 247–63

Perrin C, Jullien V, Padovani B, et al (1999) Percutaneous vertebroplasty complicated by pulmonary embolus of acrylic cement. Rev Mal Respir 16: 215–17

Ware JE Jr, Sherbourne CD (1992) The MOS 36-item short-form health survey (SF-36). I. Conceptual framework and item selection. Med Care 30(6): 473–83

Wetzel SG, Martin JB, Somon T, Wilhelm K, Rufenacht DA (2002) Painful osteolytic metastasis of the atlas: treatment with percutaneous vertebroplasty. Spine 27(22): 493–5

Microsurgical interlaminary balloon kyphoplasty

B. Boszczyk and M. Bierschneider

Interlaminary balloon kyphoplasty is a microsurgical variation of the open bipedicular technique described by Wenger and Markwalder [1999]. This access has been used previously in patients with an extensive posterior wall fracture and/or with neural compression symptoms [Boszczyk 2004].

This microsurgical operation is performed under general anesthesia. The positioning of the patient corresponds to the normal knee-chest positioning in microsurgical discectomy or decompression. The projection of the interlaminar gap on the posterior wall of the vertebra is chosen as the point to access the affected vertebra. If two adjacent vertebral bodies have to be treated, the joint interlaminar gap should be chosen. In general, only one side, the side causing the trouble, should be accessed. A symptomatic dissection of the thoracolumbar fascia is carried out via a median approx. 5 cm incision of the skin. The paravertebral muscles are pushed aside and the interlaminar space is exposed. While carefully sparing the neural structures, a lateral excision of the flaval ligament and a laminotomy are performed, exposing the lateral margin of the dural sac. Depending on the neural symptoms, a decompression is carried out laterally, in a joint-sparing manner, and carefully expanded to the opposite side by undercutting. After complete decompression, the dural sac is carefully mobilized medially and the posterior wall of the affected vertebral body is visualized (Fig. 49). The working trocar is introduced through this posterior wall with slight hammer blows towards the mid-line of the anterior wall. Compression of the neural structures must be avoided. Now a single kyphoplasty balloon is introduced via the operating cannula and brought into a central position (Fig. 51). In general it will be possible to carry out the described techniques in the area of the lumbar spine and the thoracolumbar transition without problems, if the spinal canal has normal width (Fig. 50). A medial pedicle resection might be necessary in the area of the middle thoracic spine. The fracture reduction and augmentation is carried out as described for the percutaneous techniques. Microsurgical balloon kyphoplasty allows immediate inspection of the spinal canal in the case of cement leakage. PMMA that has escaped can usually be removed without problems before hardening as it does not adhere to the dura.

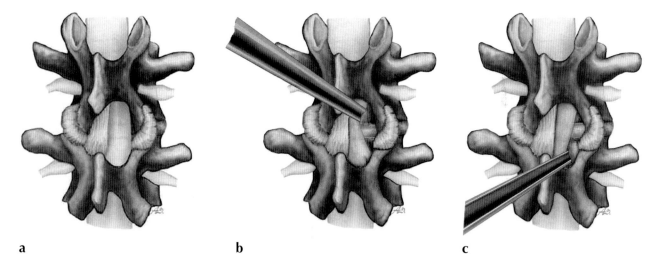

Fig. 49. a–c Dorsal view of a motion segment after interlaminary fenestration with flavectomy on the right-hand side (**a**). Presentation of the access point (**b**) at the posterior wall of the upper vertebral body by mobilization of the neural structures. Presentation of the access point (**c**) at the posterior wall of the lower vertebral body by mobilization of the neural structures

Microsurgical interlaminary balloon kyphoplasty

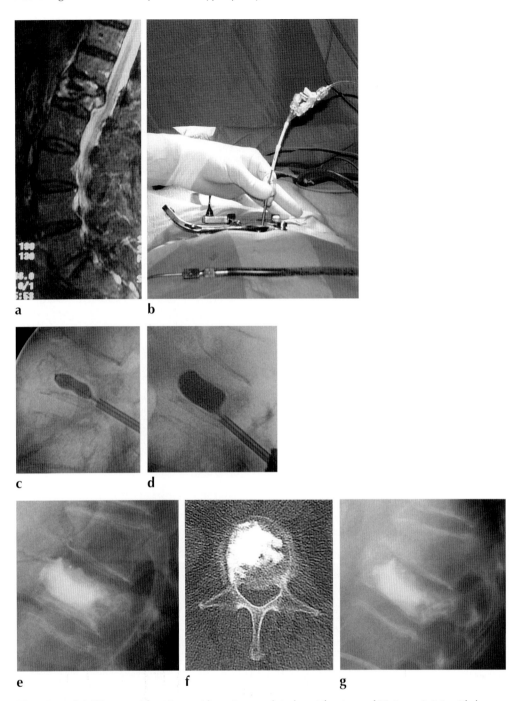

Fig. 50. a–f A 79-year-old patient with an incomplete burst fracture of L1 type A 3.1 with large posterior wall fragment and substantial loss of height after falling and several weeks of unsuccessful conservative treatment (**a**) [Boszczyk 2002]. An interlaminar access allows secure placing of the kyphoplasty balloon in the vertebral body (**b**). The lateral X-ray shows a subtotal fracture reduction by inflation of a single kyphoplasty balloon (**c–d**). The augmentation result shows acceptable filling of the vertebral body in the anterior and medial third of the vertebral body (**e, f**). The operation lasted 70 minutes, the loss of blood was 120 ml. 18 months after the operation a partial height loss can be detected with ventral spondylophyte formation, and satisfactory reduction of pain caused by the fracture (**g**)

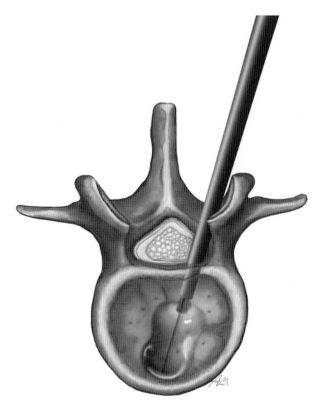

Fig. 51. End position of kyphoplasty balloon that was introduced into the vertebral body centrally at the posterior wall

References

Boszczyk B, Bierschneider M, Potulski M, Robert B, Vastmans J, Jaksche H (2002) Erweitertes Anwendungsspektrum der Kyphoplastie zur Stabilisierung der osteoporotischen Wirbelfraktur. Unfallchirurg 105: 952–7

Boszczyk BM, Bierschneider M, Schmid K, Grillhösl A, Robert B, Jaksche H (2004) Microsurgical interlaminary vertebro- and kyphoplasty for severe osteoporotic fractures. J Neurosurg 100: 32–7

Wenger W, Markwalder TM (1999) Surgically controlled, transpedicular methyl methacrylate vertebroplasty with flouroscopic guidance. Acta Neurochir (Wien) 141: 625–31

Special balloon kyphoplasty techniques in cases of screw loosening and in spinal defects

S. Becker and M. Ogon

If traumatic fractures of the spine are operated, they are primarily stabilized with an internal fixator. Complications with loosening of the pedicle screws particularly occur in patients with osteoporosis, with reported loosening rates of up to 11% [Dickman 1992; Essens 1993]. Internal fixation fails more often in an osteoporotic spine because the stability is directly dependent on the bone quality [von Strempel 1994; Wittenberg 1991]. In the following we describe four kyphoplastic techniques that can be used in cases of instrumentation failure, in older patients with osteoporosis and in spinal defects (egg-shell technique).

Transpedicular balloon kyphoplasty after screw removal (Fig. 52)

In transpedicular balloon kyphoplasty the dislocated screw is removed in a regular open procedure. The operating cannula can then be introduced transpedicularly without problems via a Kirschner wire. The only difficulty here is the fixation of the operating cannula: because the screw will also have caused a pedicle defect in most cases, the operating cannula must be manually fixed if inflating the balloon with more than 2 ml, as otherwise the balloon will have the tendency to dislocate dorsally, possibly leading eventually to a defect of the posterior wall. This complication has not yet occurred with any of our patients. However, it is advisable, as soon as the operating cannula is placed on one side, to insert the balloon kyphoplasty catheter and to inflate the balloon up to approx. 0.5 ml, as this fixes the operating cannula and thus there is no danger of the operating cannula slipping ipsilaterally when the contralateral access is performed.

Another problem arises, associated with the risk of cement leakage: screw loosening generally leads to perforation of the end plate and the adjacent basal lamina may be eroded. This means that a considerable defect can occur, reaching into the adjacent vertebra. During balloon kyphoplasty, there is the possibility of cement leaking into this large defect and therefore special attention should be paid to the viscosity of the cement (s. chapter 7).

In addition, the egg-shell technique (see below) is indicated in these cases.

Augmentation techniques (Fig. 53)

Balloon kyphoplasty can be optimally used as a ventral support for screw augmentation, if biomechanical considerations call for an extension of the instrumentation or if the bone is so osteoporotic that screw loosening is very likely and stabilization with an internal fixator is inevitable. Normal balloon kyphoplasty is performed on the vertebra before the augmentation is carried out. The osteointroducer must be removed before the cement hardens, as the screws have to be brought into the still soft cement; once the cement has hardened, it can be difficult or even impossible to apply the screws properly, as a hole would then have to be drilled into the cement, and an appropriate bony support is often missing ventrally. Furthermore, it should be noted that vertebrae adjacent to the fixation have a very high risk of spontaneous fractures, therefore prophylactic stabilization is always indicated here.

The egg-shell technique (Fig. 54)

In cases of large vertebral defects the so-called egg-shell technique is helpful. A PMMA lining is erected in the area of the vertebral wall defect by first bringing in 0.5 ml of low-viscosity cement, followed by the balloon catheter and inflation of the balloon. High-viscosity cement may disrupt the balloon as a consequence of the chemical binding heat of the cement. The inflation causes the balloon to squeeze the cement into the wall defect, by which the egg shell, i.e. the PMMA wall, is created. After removing the balloon catheter the cement can be applied in the usual consistency; this reduces the risk of extravazation considerably. This technique should be used under all circumstances after a screw removal, especially if the screws have caused large defects extending into the next vertebra. Cement that has been applied in this manner has considerably less tendency to leak from the vertebral body; however, leakage cannot always be avoided in cases of larger defects after screw loosening.

Support technique (Fig. 55)

This technique is helpful if an open operation with removal of screws is no longer possible. In the support technique the balloon is brought into the vertebra adjacent to the vertebra with the loosened

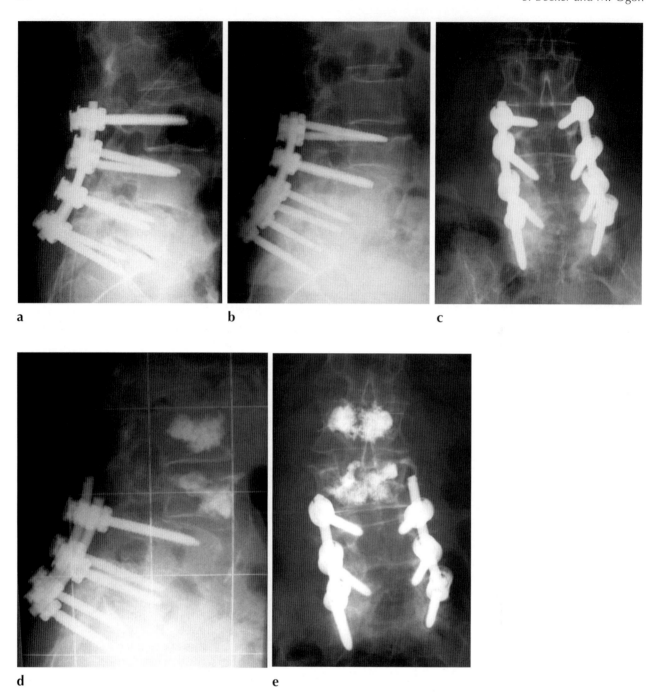

Fig. 52. Balloon kyphoplasty after screw removal. A 78-year-old female patient with an absolute spinal stenosis of L3/L4 and of L4/L5, which was decompressed and stabilized primarily at the level of L3–S1 (**a**). A routine check after 3 months revealed loosening of the screws of L3, without the patient showing any symptoms of pain (**b**, **c**). Because of this loosening, the L3 screws were removed, the longitudinal rod was cut correspondingly, and a transpedicular balloon kyphoplasty carried out using the above technique at the level of L3, as well as a prophylactic balloon kyphoplasty at the level of L2 (**d**, **e**)

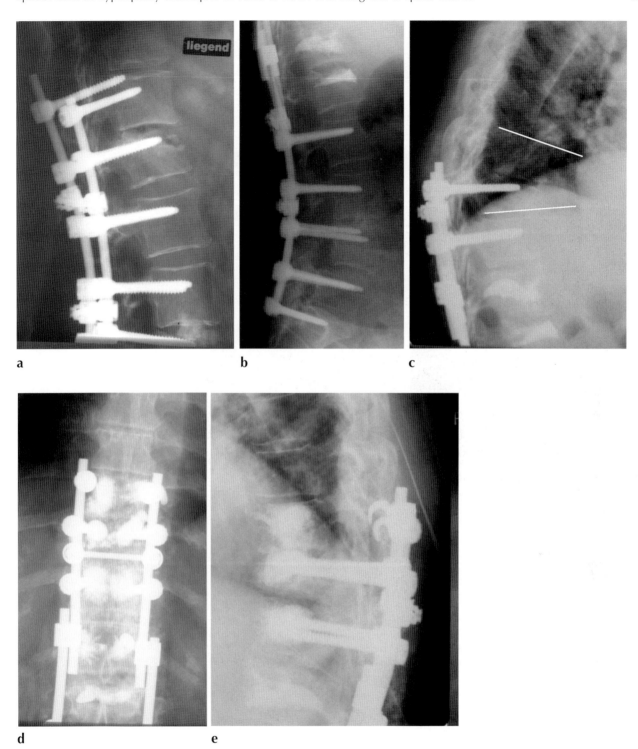

Fig. 53. See Fig. 54

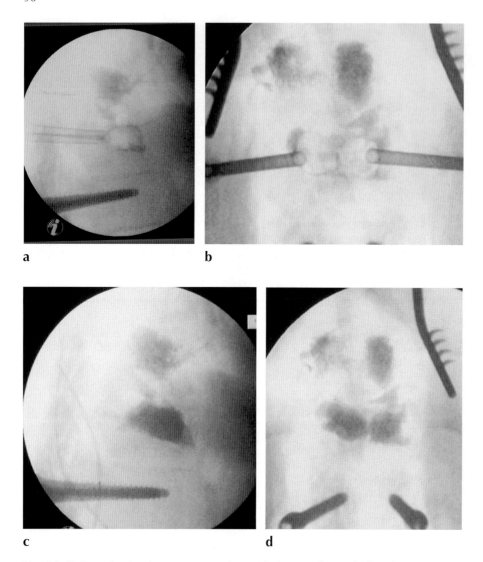

Fig. 54. Balloon kyphoplasty augmentation technique and egg shell technique. A 60-year-old female patient with severe degenerative scoliosis of the lumbar spine, which was dorsally instrumented from T12 to S1 and restored scoliosis. After a fall the screws of the segment T12 and L1 came loose (**Fig. 53a**), therefore balloon kyphoplasty was performed on these segments and the instrumentation was prolonged to T10 (**Fig. 53b**, **c**). 4 weeks after this operation the cranial screws of T10 and T11 came loose again (**Fig. 53c**); this time the screws of T10 and T11 had to be augmented with balloon kyphoplasty as well as the eroded basal lamina of T9 (**Fig. 53d**, **e**). For further stabilization with a longer lever arm, an additional fixation of segment T9 was carried out using transversal hooks of the fracture system (USS®, Synthes). Because of the big defect/damage of T10, the egg shell technique was used on both sides before introduction of the screws (**Fig. 54**). This reduced the cement leakage considerably

screws. It is important that the balloon lies at the affected endplate, i.e. in most cases in the direction of the basal endplate. If any screws penetrate here, a screw can be used as a support to inflate the balloon in a cranial direction and thus correct the kyphotic malposition again. Alternatively a unidirectional balloon can be used.

Use of the balloon kyphoplasty techniques described above has advantages in cases of revision, screw loosening and augmentation. Augmentation of screws has already been performed with PMMA cement for some time, but until now with a vertebroplasty [Steffee 1986, 1988; Zucherman 1988]. The augmentation considerably improves the pullout strength of the screws [von Strempel 1994]. Once a balloon catheter has been used to stabilize a vertebra, it can be easily reused on adjacent segments to reinforce the screws in order to avoid leakage.

We perform balloon kyphoplasty in cases of loosening of the internal fixator as an operative stabilization method. Using the techniques described above, we have several possible methods at our disposal for stabilization of the spine, without having to extend the instrumentation proximally or distally. This reduces the operation time and risk of infection considerably. In our opinion conservative therapy is not indicated in cases of screw loosening or for osteoporotic fractures either above or below the implant, as an increase of the malposition of the spine is likely because of the different elastic qualities of the implant and the fractured vertebra. A critical point regarding our operation methods is that, despite the egg-shell technique and the optimal cementing technique, leakage of cement into surrounding tissues cannot always be prevented. Moreover, depending on the kind of fracture, optimal restoration of the kyphosis cannot always be achieved, so that in these rare operations, which should be considered as rescue operations in difficult cases, primary stability with early mobilization and relief of pain surely have priority.

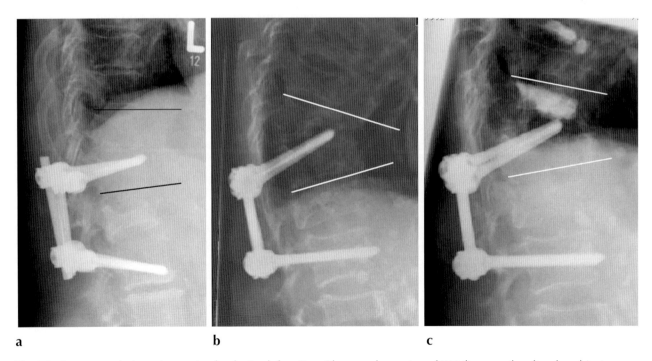

Fig. 55. Support technique: Increasing kyphotic deformity with screw loosening of T12 five months after dorsal instrumentation of an L1 fracture in a 72-year-old female patient (**a**, **b**). Because of internal accompanying diseases, an open operation with screw removal was not possible and therefore balloon kyphoplasty was only carried out on the fractured vertebra T11. The balloon was positioned directly on the loosened screw, using it as a support for the restoration of the kyphosis. The screw was left in situ and therefore, as expected, there was no leakage of cement (**c**). The patient could be mobilized the following day, and findings were stable in the 6 month follow-up, without any pain problems

References

Dickman C, Fessler RG, MacMillan M, et al (1992) Transpedicular screw-rod fixation of the lumbar spine: operative technique and outcome in 104 cases. J Neurosurg 77: 860–70

Essens S, Sacs BL, Drezyin V (1993) Complications associated with the technique of pedicle screw fixation: a selected survey of ABC members. Spine 18: 2231–9

Steffee AD, Sitkowski DJ, Topham LS (1986) Total vertebral body and pedicle arthroplasty. Clin Orthop Relat R 203: 203–8

Steffee AD, Sitkowsky DJ (1988) Reduction and stabilization of grade IV spondylolisthesis. Clin Orthop Relat R 227: 82–9

von Strempel A, Kühle J, Plitz W (1994) Stabilität von Pedikelschrauben. Teil 2: Maximale Auszugskräfte unter Berücksichtigung der Knochendichte. Z Orthop 132: 82–6

von Strempel A, Seidel T, Plitz W (1994) Stabilität von Pedikelschrauben. Teil 1: Maximale Auszugskräfte bei knochengesunden Stammwirbelsäulen unter Berücksichtigung der Bohrtechnik. Z Orthop 132: 75–81

Wittenberg RH, Shea M, Swartz DE, Lee KS, White III AA, Hayes WC (1991) Importance of bone mineral density in instrumented spine fusions. Spine 16: 647–52

Zucherman J, Hsu K, White A, Wynne G (1988) Early results of spinal fusion using variable spine plating system. Spine 13: 570–9

The treatment of vertebral osteonecrosis and vertebra plana with balloon kyphoplasty

S. Becker

Although conservative treatment is generally regarded as the gold standard in osteoporotic vertebral fractures, it carries the risk of advanced vertebral collapse, increased kyphosis and persisting pain (Figs. 56, 58). Those severe collapses may result in vertebra plana fractures, which are usually difficult to treat and are generally a contraindication for percutaneous techniques. However, it has been reported that cases with pseudarthrosis, osteonecrosis or fluid/gas signs on X-ray/MRI are treatable with vertebroplasty [Huy 1998; Jang 2003].

Osteonecrosis has been reported in several different bones, and in the spine this disease has various names: osteonecrosis, vascular necrosis, pseudarthrosis and Kümmel's spondylitis [Chou 1997; Hasegawa 1998; Huy 1998; Ito 2005; Jang 2003; Maheshwari 2004; Murakami 2003]. All these descriptions may simply be different names for the same disease, the most non-specific description being "Kümmel or Kümmel-Verneuil spondylitis", which is based on a case series from 1895 [Van Eenenaam 1993, Young 2002]. All the descriptions have the same findings on X-ray and MRI. On X-Ray or CT we typically find an intravertebral cleft, also described as a "gas sign" demonstrating fluid and gas in the intravertebral body [Bhalla 1998; McKiernan and Faciszewski 2003] (Figs. 56–58). This sign is typically benign and does not warrant biopsy [Bhalla 1998]. On MRI we find fluid or gas in the vertebral body; this can be seen as a dark zone on T1 and bright on T2/STIR [Hasegawa 1998; Maheshwari 2004; McKiernan and Faciszewski 2003] (Fig. 58). These findings typically persist as long as the fracture remains unhealed and shows clinical instability, with a high risk of further progression into a vertebra plana (Figs. 56, 58) or development of severe kyphosis (Fig. 56).

The different descriptions also all have the same histological findings, such as necrotic granulation and fatty degeneration of the bone tissue, and a fibrocartilaginous membrane surrounding the fluid with the absence of any new endochondral bone [Antonacci 2002; Hasegawa 1998; Murakami 2003].

Clinically, several risk factors can cause osteonecrosis: malignancy, infection, radiation therapy, liver

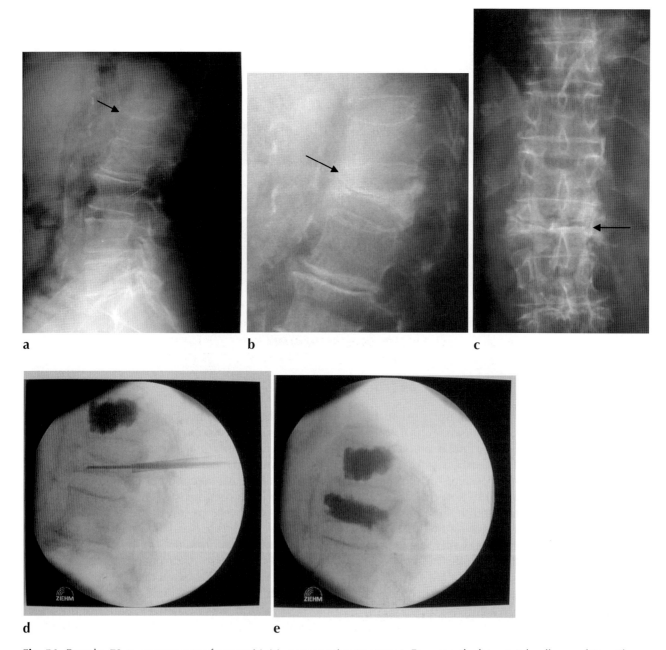

Fig. 56. Female, 72 y., spontaneous fracture L1 (**a**), conservative treatment. Four months later, total collapse of L1 with osteonecrosis (**b**). Intraoperative reduction on OR table with k-wire in place and prophylactic adjacent stabilization (**c**) and result after balloon kyphoplasty (**d**)

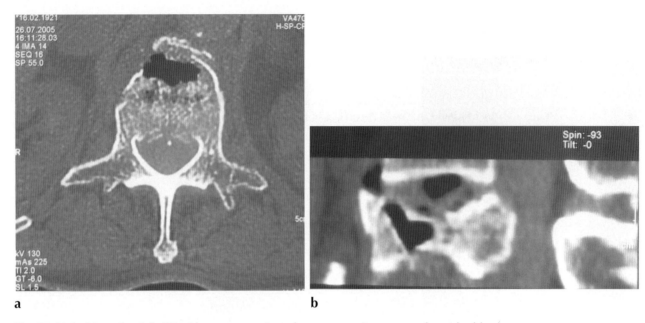

Fig. 57. Male 84 y, after fall, CT with osteonecrosis and gas on anterior aspect of vertebral body

cirrhosis, alcoholism, steroid treatments [Allen 1987; Brower 1981; Chou 1997; Lieberman 2001; Maldague 1978; Van Bockel 1987], rarely sarcoidosis [Ito 2005], hemoglobinopathies such as sickle cell anemia [Maheshwari 2004], Cushing syndrome and Gaucher syndrome [Ito 2005], and dysbarism after diving accidents [Hutter 2000]. In trauma it has been postulated that disruption of the anterior vessels may cause osteonecrosis, which explains why osteonecrosis is found anteriorly in some cases (Fig. 57).

This dynamic instability of osteonecrotic vertebral fractures [McKiernan and Jensen 2003] is persistent with chronic pain and is the main clinical finding. The instability can be typically seen with the patient in a prone position either on the X-Ray table or in the OR (Figs. 56, 59) and is a valuable sign that balloon kyphoplasty is feasible, because the partial closed reduction of the fracture, due to the positioning, facilitates the insertion of the balloon kyphoplasty tools. In cases of uncertainty regarding osteonecrosis on X-ray (Figs. 59, 60), we favor a prone X-ray rather than a CT, because it demonstrates the reduction capability better and can be done in any radiological facility.

Whatever may be the cause of vertebral collapse and osteonecrosis, surgical treatment with vertebroplasty or balloon kyphoplasty is uniform. In general, osteonecrosis has poor capacity to heal, but the dynamic instability that causes the symptoms can be alleviated by cementoplasty. In the literature, good results have been reported in osteonecrosis patients with vertebroplasty [Huy 1998; Jang 2003]. We retrospectively reviewed our balloon kyphoplasties on vertebra plana fractures from 2002 to 2005, during which period we performed 230 balloon kyphoplasties on 139 patients. The retrospective analysis showed a complete collapse with vertebra plana in 15 patients (mean age 76 years, SD 5.2 years, 3 male, 12 female) and osteonecrosis signs in eight patients. The pre- and postoperative vertebral height (anterior, middle and posterior heights) and the kyphotic angle are shown in Table 8. The average time of postoperative surgical treatment was eight weeks after the fracture (9.62 weeks in the osteonecrosis group, 6.14 weeks in the vertebra plana group). The treated vertebrae were Th7 and Th9 (1 case each), Th11 and Th12 (2 cases each), L2 (3 cases) and L1 (6 cases].

Our results (Table 8) show more significant restoration of the vertebral height after balloon kyphoplasty in the osteonecrosis group than in the vertebroplasty group ($p < 0.013$). Correction of the kyphotic angle was achieved in both groups but was

The treatment of vertebral osteonecrosis and vertebra plana with balloon kyphoplasty

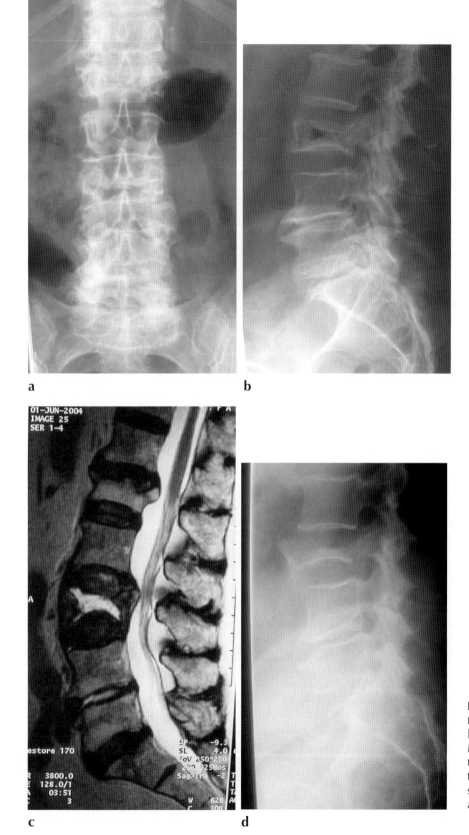

Fig. 58. Female, 85 y., spontaneous fracture L3 with osteonecrosis, clearly visible on the lateral X-ray (**b**). The MRI also shows fluid within the vertebral body (**c**). Five months later after conservative treatment, severe segmental collapse with chronic pain and immobility (**d**)

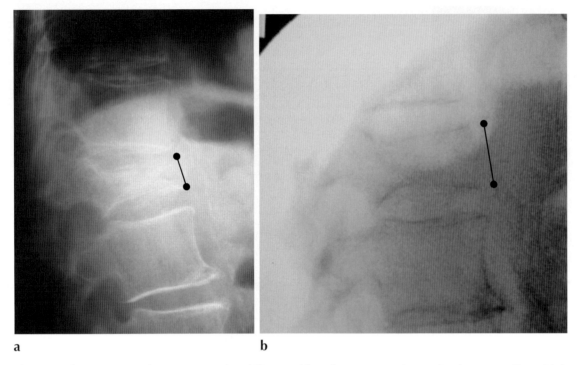

Fig. 59. Male, 84 y., typical osteonecrotic instability L1, although osteonecrosis not clearly seen on X-ray (**a**), but total reduction of fracture 4 weeks after onset of pain in prone position on OR table (**b**)

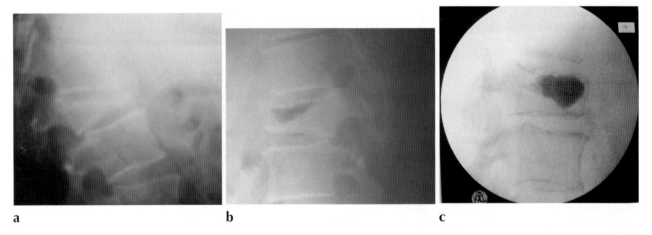

Fig. 60. Male, 72 y. fracture L1 with uncertain sign of osteonecrosis (**a**). The instability assessment in the prone position clearly shows gas in the vertebra and a good closed reduction of the fracture (**b**). The postoperative image after balloon kyphoplasty still shows an increase in vertebral height (**c**)

The treatment of vertebral osteonecrosis and vertebra plana with balloon kyphoplasty 103

Table 8. Mean correction of kyphotic angle, anterior vertebral height (AH), middle vertebral height (MH) and posterior vertebral height (PH) in the osteonecrosis and vertebra plana groups

	Osteonecrosis group – mean	Vertebra plana group – mean	p-values
Kyphosis post-op	10,375° SD 6,89	3,71° SD 4,42	p = 0.099
AH	33,095%* SD 13,55	4.92% SD 4,57	p < 0.001*
MH	37,835%* SD 12,76	17.51% SD 9,42	p = 0.004*
PH	19,076%* SD 18,08	1.83% SD 2,58	p = 0.031*

*Statistically significant difference.

not significant, because a vertebra plana without any kyphotic component very often does not cause kyphotic deformity of the whole spine.

Comparing our data with the literature, it seems that in our series of complicated cases with advanced vertebral collapse the correction capacity of balloon kyphoplasty is superior to the capacity in "normal" osteoporotic fractures [Garfin 2001; Ledlie 2003; Theodorou 2002]. The latter authors all described the balloon kyphoplasty procedure on osteoporotic vertebral fractures and reported a correction of the vertebral height between 8% and 20%.

The clinical outcome of our two groups combined showed the following: the physical component summary score (PCSS) improved from 27.3 preoperatively to 36.2 postoperatively, as did the mental component summary score (MCSS; pre-op 33.35, post-op 41), Oswestry score (pre-op 64.3, post-op 46.5) and the VAS (pre-op 6.8, post-op 4.2). There was no statistical difference in clinical outcome between the two groups. The results show significant improvement of the PCSS, Oswestry score and VAS in both groups, which has been well reported after vertebroplasty and balloon kyphoplasty. The fact that both groups showed postoperative improvement, basically independent of whether osteonecrosis was apparent or not, supports the indication for minimally invasive stabilization of vertebral fractures with cement, even if corrections of height or kyphosis cannot be achieved.

In conclusion, in osteonecrosis there is a high risk of severe collapse and early intervention is required. Balloon kyphoplasty and vertebroplasty can significantly improve the vertebral height and major changes of the kyphotic angle are possible. Even after several months, correction of the deformity is possible with balloon kyphoplasty. Nevertheless, all patients with a positive fracture sign are treatable with cementoplasty to alleviate their pain.

References

Allen BL Jr, Jinkins WJ 3rd (1987) Vertebral osteonecrosis associated with pancreatitis in a child. A case report. J Bone Joint Surg Am 60(7): 985–7

Antonacci MD, Mody DR, Rutz K, Weilbaecher D, Heggeness MH (2002) A histologic study of fractured human vertebral bodies. Journal of Spinal Disorders & Techniques 15(2): 118–26

Bhalla S, Reinus WR (1998) The linear intravertebral vacuum: a sign of benign vertebral collapse. Am J Roentgenol 170(6): 1563–9

Brower AC, Downey EF Jr (1981) Kummell disease: report of a case with serial radiographs. Radiology 141(2): 363–4

Chou LH, Knight RQ (1997) Idiopathic avascular necrosis of a vertebral body. Case report and literature review. Spine 22(16): 1928–32

Garfin SR, Yuan HA, Reiley MA (2001) New technologies in spine: kyphoplasty and vertebroplasty for the treatment of painful osteoporotic compression fractures. Spine 26(14): 1511–5

Hasegawa K, Homma T, Uchiyama S, Takahashi H (1998) Vertebral pseudarthrosis in the osteoporotic spine. Spine 23(20): 2201–6

Hutter CD (2000) Dysbaric osteonecrosis: a reassessment and hypothesis. Med Hypotheses 54(4): 585–90

Huy MD, Jensen ME, Marx WF, Kallmes DF (1998) Percutaneous vertebroplasty in vertebral osteonecrosis (Kümmell's spondylitis). Neurosurg Focus (1), Article 2 (online journal)

Ito M, Motomiya M, Abumi K, Shirado O, Kotani Y, Kadoya K, Murota E, Minami A (2005) Vertebral osteonecrosis associated with sarcoidosis. Case report. J Neurosurg Spine 2(2): 222–5

Jang JS, Kim DY, Lee SH (2003) Efficacy of percutaneous vertebroplasty in the treatment of intravertebral pseudarthrosis associated with noninfected avascular necrosis of the vertebral body. Spine 28(14): 1588–92

Ledlie JT, Renfro M (20039 Balloon kyphoplasty: one-year outcomes in vertebral body height restoration, chronic pain and activity levels. J Neurosurg Spine 98 [1 Suppl]: 36–42

Lieberman IH, Dudeney S, Reinhardt MK, Bell G (2001) Initial outcome and efficacy of kyphoplasty in the treatment of painful osteoporotic vertebral compression fractures. Spine 26(14): 1631–8

Maheshwari PR, Nagar AM, Prasad SS, Shah JR, Patkar DP (2004) Avascular necrosis of spine: a rare appearance. Spine 29(6): 119–22

Maldague BE, Noel HM, Malghem JJ (1978) The intravertebral vacuum cleft: a sign of ischemic vertebral collapse. Radiology 129(1): 23–9

McKiernan F, Faciszewski T (2003) Intravertebral clefts in osteoporotic vertebral compression fractures. Arthritis Rheum 48(5): 1414–9

McKiernan F, Jensen R, Faciszewski T (2003) The dynamic mobility of vertebral compression fractures. J Bone & Mineral Res 18: 24–9

Murakami H, Kawahara N, Gabata T, Nambu K, Tomita K (2003) Vertebral body osteonecrosis without vertebral collapse. Spine 28(16): 323–8

Theodorou DJ, Theodorou SJ, Duncan TD, Garfin SR, Wong WH (2002) Percutaneous balloon kyphoplasty for the correction of spinal deformity in painful vertebral body compression fractures. Clin Imaging 26(1): 1–5

Van Bockel SR, Mindelzun RE (1987) Gas in the psoas muscle secondary to an intravertebral vacuum cleft: CT characteristics. J Comput Assist Tomogr 11(5): 913–5

Van Eenenaam DP, el-Khoury GY (1993) Delayed post-traumatic vertebral collapse (Kummell's disease): case report with serial radiographs, computed tomographic scans, and bone scans. Spine 18(9): 1236–41

Young WF, Brown D, Kendler A, Clements D (2002) Delayed post-traumatic osteonecrosis of a vertebral body (Kummell's disease). Acta Orthop Belg 68(1): 13–9

Chapter 10

Indications and experience with balloon kyphoplasty in trauma

The safety and treatment possibilities of balloon kyphoplasty have rapidly led to the use of this technique in traumatic vertebral fractures. Initially balloon kyphoplasty was used in osteoporotic patients who sustained a fall and a subsequent traumatic fracture; however, the general rules of balloon kyphoplasty also apply in trauma cases and the guidelines shown above remain valid. Although we now have a safe and effective method of restoring vertebral height and reducing the fracture, the injectable bone substance is still an issue, especially in trauma. In general there is consensus that polymethylmethacrylate (PMMA) is safer in the elderly, as it is not resorbed or remodeled, but in young patients consensus has not yet been found on whether the use of PMMA in traumatic fracture is safe. During the past five years resorbable calcium phosphate cements (CPC) have therefore gained in popularity. In this chapter we summarize knowledge of the use of balloon kyphoplasty with resorbable CPC in traumatic fractures in young patients.

Balloon-assisted endplate reduction combined with vertebroplasty for the treatment of traumatic vertebral body fractures

J.-J. Verlaan, W. J. A. Dhert, and
F. Cumhur Oner

Current approaches and techniques for the treatment of traumatic vertebral fractures

The optimal treatment of traumatic thoracolumbar fractures has, in the absence of properly conducted trials, been fiercely debated and, despite numerous publications showing lower levels of evidence in the past four decades, no consensus currently exists [Thomas 2006; Verlaan and Diekerhof 2004; Wood 2003]. Most spine surgeons will agree that the majority of A.1 and A.2 fractures (according to the AO classification by Magerl et al.) can be treated without operative intervention; A.3 fractures sometimes require surgery and B-type or C-type fractures almost always require surgery for good outcome [Magerl 1984; Vaccaro 2005]. Some discussions in the literature have focused on the best surgical approach for fracture reduction and fixation. In a recent systematic review of the literature it was noted that scientific evidence does not favor any particular surgical approach and preferences are most likely to be based on personal or institutional experiences [Thomas 2006; Verlaan and Diekerhof 2004]. It can be concluded from the literature that posterior short-segment fixation is currently the easiest surgical technique with relatively minor complications and generating good-to-excellent results in the majority of cases [Korovessis 2006; Verlaan and Diekerhof 2004]. However, for some fractures, especially complete vertebral body burst fractures (A.3.3), posterior short-segment fixation has sometimes been noted to be less successful [McCormack 1994]. In a radiological investigation of cadaveric traumatic fractures by Oner et al., it was hypothesized that some types of disk space disruption may result from the traumatic impact and can subsequently lead to secondary kyphosis as a consequence of disk subsidence through the fractured endplate into the vertebral body [Oner 1998]. Radiological observations of clinical cases correlated with these experimental findings that changes in disk space morphology often result after traumatic fractures [Oner 1999]. Furthermore, in fractures apparently sufficiently reduced on initial radiographs, it was shown that recurrent kyphosis may occur as a result of intervertebral disk intrusion into the burst vertebral body [Oner 1998]. A study by Speth et al. subsequently confirmed these findings in a cohort of patients with traumatic burst fractures treated with posterior reduction and fixation [Speth 1995]. It was demonstrated in a series of experimental studies that disk space redistribution resulting from intrusion into the vertebral body could be prevented by proper endplate reduction and intravertebral augmentation of the resulting sub-endplate void [Verlaan 2002]. The technique for achieving endplate reduction was by direct reduction with inflatable bone tamps and injection of CPC. The studies that led to the procedure for fractured endplate reduction and vertebral body augmentation are the topic of the current chapter.

Experimental and clinical studies for the development of transpedicular augmentation techniques of the anterior spinal column in traumatic fractures

First steps in developing a direct reduction technique for burst fractures

In 1999 the authors developed the concept of using balloons for endplate reduction in traumatic burst type fractures (balloon-assisted endplate reduction, BAER), combined with vertebroplasty (VTP). The predominant safety concerns were potential displacement of bone fragments towards the spinal canal after expansion of the inflatable bone tamps and subsequent leakage of cement in the spinal canal through the damaged posterior vertebral body wall. It was postulated that primary reduction of the burst fracture by ligamentotaxis and subsequent fixation with a rigid pedicle screw construct would prevent this displacement. The technique was first tested in a human cadaveric fracture model [Verlaan 2002]. Traumatic burst fractures were created in 23 non-osteoporotic thoracolumbar specimens. The frac-

tures were reduced using short-segment pedicle screw constructs, and the endplates were subsequently reduced using transpedicularly introduced inflatable bone tamps (KyphX, Kyphon Inc.). The cavities that resulted after deflation and removal of the balloons were filled with CPC (BoneSource®, Stryker Orthopedics) consisting of equimolar amounts of dicalcium and tetracalcium phosphate which, when mixed with saline, form hydroxyapatite. Plain radiographs (anteroposterior and lateral) and magnetic resonance images (MRIs) were obtained from the specimens after fracturing, after reduction and posterior stabilization, and after the BAER/VTP procedure. Distraction of the fractures by pedicle screw instrumentation resulted in a reduction of both anterior and posterior wall displacement but did not reduce the central impression of the fractured endplate, probably because of persistent hydrostatic intervertebraldisk pressure. After BAER and VTP the impression of the central endplate was significantly decreased. See also Fig. 61 for a chronological series of fluoroscopical images obtained during the experimental procedure. The maximum posterior wall displacement caused by BAER was 1.3 mm. No cement leakage outside the vertebral body could be detected during the procedure or after examination of the sectioned specimens. It was concluded that BAER and VTP might be safely used as a less invasive technique for anterior column reconstruction for selected burst-type fractures.

The choice of cement as a bone-void filler. An animal model for vertebroplasty

After optimal reduction of the fractured endplates with BAER, the ensuing cavity in the vertebral body should be filled with a material strong enough to resist the hydrostatic expansive force from the adjacent disks, and preferably not interfere with fracture healing. Autologous bone could be used, but experience with transpedicular spongioplasty as additional treatment to posterior fixation suggests that graft necrosis frequently develops [Alanay 2001; Verlaan and Diekerhof 2004]. Furthermore, crushed bone may not be strong enough when used for this application. Traditionally, PMMA cement has been used successfully for vertebroplasty in osteoporotic compression fractures [Heini 2000]; however, it might not be a good idea to inject PMMA cement into fresh traumatic fractures, as its permanent presence between bone fragments would preclude bone

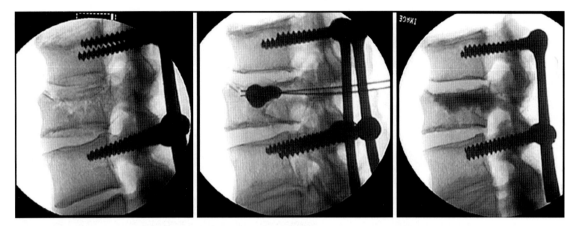

Fig. 61. Chronological series of fluoroscopic images demonstrating the procedure of balloon vertebroplasty for traumatic fractures after posterior fixation in a human cadaveric thoracolumbar specimen

healing. Furthermore, if extracorporal leakage of cement has occurred, exothermic polymerization of PMMA cement could lead to thermal damage of vulnerable neurovascular structures, although some publications on this topic suggest the chances of serious complications resulting from heat necrosis to be low [Aebli 2006; Belkoff 2003; Deramond 1999; Verlaan 2003]. CPC, already used with good results as bone-void filler in the treatment of distal radius and tibial plateau fractures, may be an interesting alternative to PMMA cement for specific vertebroplasty applications [Nakano 2002 and 2005]. Since we can expect direct contact of bone cement with disk tissue in acute traumatic endplate fractures, not only the effects on bone healing but also effects on the viability of intervertebral disk tissue become important. These biocompatibility issues were studied in an *in vivo* goat model described below [Verlaan and Oner 2004].

In two vertebral bodies (L3 and L5) of the lumbar spine of 24 goats, cavities were created by drilling and reaming through a transpedicular approach (Fig. 62). In half of the treated vertebral bodies a defect was also drilled in the cranial endplate to allow for direct contact between cement and nucleus pulposus. The cavities were filled with either PMMA cement (Simplex®, Stryker Corporation) or CPC (BoneSource®, Stryker Corporation) according to assignment to one of four groups: vertebroplasty with CPC with or without cranial endplate defect; vertebroplasty with PMMA cement with or without cranial endplate defect (Fig. 63). Another six goats from unrelated research were used as controls. The follow-up periods were six weeks and six months. The postmortem intervertebral disks, endplates and surrounding tissues were examined with semiquantitative histological analysis and radiography.

In none of the animals were radiological or histological signs of disk degeneration seen, supporting clinical observations that isolated central endplate defects/fractures do not consistently cause disk degeneration, although this finding may well be different in displaced fractures and disrupted disks. In all

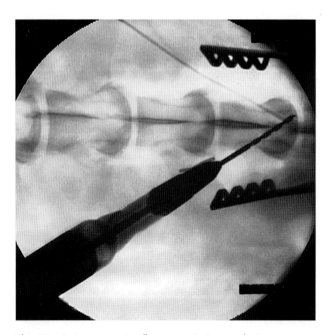

Fig. 62. Anteroposterior fluoroscopic image during transpedicular drilling of the goat vertebral body

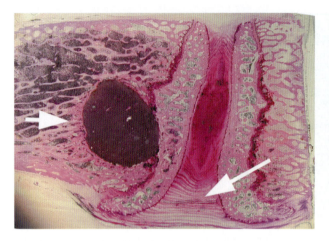

Fig. 63. Low magnification photograph of a histological section demonstrating a goat spine segment (cranial vertebral body-dish-caudal vertebral body) six weeks after calcium phosphate cement (CPC) vertebroplasty. The arrows point to excellent osseointegration of CPC and intact lamellar configuration of the annulus fibrosus

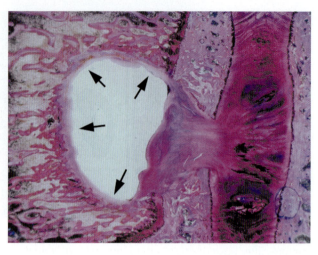

Fig. 64. Low magnification photograph of a histological section six weeks after PMMA vertebroplasty including an endplate defect to allow for nucleus pulposus-cement contact. The arrows point to the fibrous tissue layer between cement and cancellous bone

PMMA specimens, regardless of contact of the cement with disk tissue, a fibrous layer was found between cement and bone (Fig. 64). In some cases a mild inflammatory reaction was observed around the PMMA cement. In the CPC specimens, histological signs of close cement-bone integration and some early remodeling were observed. Although recent (yet unpublished) observations by others describe lethal complications after intentional extravasation of CPC in an animal model, no peri- or postoperative problems were encountered in our cohort of goats [Bernhard 2003].

This study indicated that for traumatic fractures, which are suffered mainly by young and active patients, CPC, because of its favorable biocompatibility, may be a more suitable bone-void filler than PMMA cement.

A clinical trial to assess the feasibility and safety of BAER and VTP for traumatic thoracolumbar fractures

Encouraged by these preclinical studies, it was decided to perform a trial in patients with burst-type fractures using BAER and VTP techniques with CPC, as an adjunct to routine posterior short-segment pedicle screw fracture reduction and fixation [Verlaan and Dhert 2005]. It was hypothesized that reducing the fractured endplate and augmenting the anterior spinal column through a transpedicular approach would decrease the chance of spine segment collapse and subsequent kyphosis, thereby decreasing the need for secondary anterior spine surgery. The clinical study proposal was approved by the institutional review board. Twenty patients, 18 years of age or older, with a recent (< 5 days) axial burst fracture (meaning A.3 and all of its subtypes, according to the AO classification) of the thoracic or lumbar spine without neurologic deficits were included after obtaining informed consent. Patients with a rupture of the posterior longitudinal ligament (PLL) on preoperative MRI examination were excluded because of safety considerations. Preoperative anteroposterior and lateral radiographs of the fractured spine were obtained, as well as MRI scans, for assessment of damage to the endplate, vertebral body and discoligamentary structures. Short-segment pedicle screw and rod reduction and fixation (Diapason®, Stryker Corporation) was performed in all cases. Using posterior instrumentation, the adjacent vertebral bodies were realigned using the conventional technique of fracture dekyphosis and distraction. The pedicles of the fractured vertebral body were subsequently identified and probed. Under fluoroscopic guidance, two cannulas were inserted into each pedicle through which KyphX balloons (Kyphon Inc.) were inserted under the fractured endplates. After positioning the balloons under the most impressed part of the endplate, using fluoroscopic

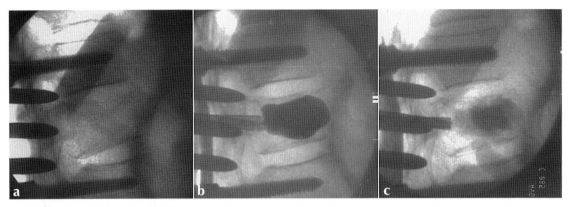

Fig. 65. Chronological series of fluoroscopic images demonstrating the clinical procedure of balloon assisted endplate reduction (BAER) with vertebroplasty (VTP) for traumatic fractures after posterior fixation: **a)** an impressed endplate even after optimal reduction of the adjacent levels; **b)** the reduction of the fractured endplate after balloon inflation; **c)** partial reduction of the endplate after balloon removal and cement injection

guidance, the bone tamps were inflated. Fluoroscopic images were obtained frequently to assess the amount of reduction achieved and to detect unwarranted (posterior) displacement of bone fragments. Subsequent individual inflation of the bone tamps allowed fine-tuning of endplate reduction and correction of asymmetric (scoliotic) deformities. The amount of CPC (BoneSource®, Stryker Corporation) needed to fill the resulting defect in the vertebral body was estimated from the total balloon volume and prepared for injection. The balloons were then deflated and removed. The defects were filled by cement injection without any pressurization under continuous fluoroscopic monitoring (Fig. 65a–c). Finally, a bisegmental posterolateral fusion with autologous iliac crest bone was performed in all cases. At approximately 17 ± 3 months follow up, the pedicle screw instrumentation was removed as part of the study protocol to evaluate the effectiveness of BAER with VTP. Anteroposterior and lateral radiographs and MRIs were obtained preoperatively, postoperatively and 1 month after removal of the posterior instrumentation. A total of 20 patients with 21 fractures were treated. No neurologic complications were encountered. Substantial correction of all radiologic parameters was observed. The average Cobb angle was corrected from 11 (± 9.2) degrees preoperatively to –1.6 (± 9.5) degrees postoperatively to 3.0 (± 11.4) degrees after instrumentation removal. The average central body height increased

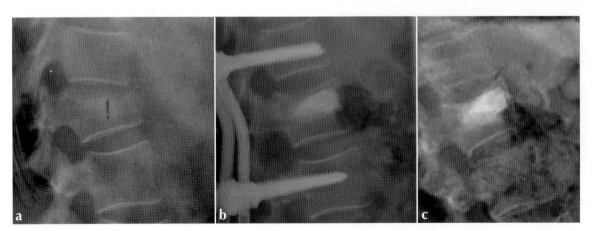

Fig. 66. Lateral radiographs of a lumbar spine showing: **a)** the initial burst fracture of L1; **b)** a good reduction after pedicle screw fixation and BAER and VTP; **c)** a good reduction one month after instrumentation removal (18 months posttrauma)

from 66% (± 10.7%) preoperatively to 81% (± 10.4%) postoperatively to 80% (± 12.0%) of the estimated intact height after instrumentation removal (Fig. 66a–c). Substantial canal clearance was observed in all cases on the sagittal MRIs at follow up. Posterior bone displacement was not detected intraoperatively or at various phases during follow up in any of the patients. Cement leakage, defined as any amount of cement outside the confines of the vertebral body, was seen in five patients. In one (asymptomatic) patient, some cement was found in the spinal canal. Although its presence in proximity of the spinal cord is highly undesirable, the longer plasticity (> 20 minutes) and isothermic curing of CPC probably makes it less hazardous at this location than PMMA cement. In the other four cases, cement leakage occurred in clinically less significant locations such as the psoas compartment twice and disk space twice. The additional BAER procedure did not cause any technical surgical difficulties and required approximately 20 minutes of extra operation time. Because we observed that early pedicle probing of the fractured vertebra caused substantial blood loss from the vertebral body, probing was postponed until after fracture reduction and instrumentation. Inflation of the balloons stopped the intravertebral bleeding immediately. It was discovered that potentially dangerous cement leakage was caused by building up (even minor) pressure in the syringe during cement injection. We subsequently developed the practice of first injecting a small amount of saline into one cannula and, when unimpeded outflow through the other cannula was observed, injection pressure could be kept low as the flow of excess cement through the contralateral cannula was unrestricted (Fig. 67). Cannula removal was also postponed until closure of the wound, allowing for initial setting of the CPC. These two practical changes resulted in no further cement leakages. Long-term follow up (> 5 years) is currently under way to study the incidence and amount of subsequent kyphosis after hardware removal.

BAER with VTP seems feasible and safe for augmentation of the anterior column in patients with selected traumatic thoracolumbar A.3 burst-type injuries. However, the superiority of this technique over nonoperative treatment or anterior/circumferential stabilization can only be reliably demonstrated with a randomized controlled study.

Detailed analysis of intraoperative changes in bone displacement and endplate reduction during balloon vertebroplasty visualized with 3D rotational X-ray imaging

Although we had shown the feasibility of BAER and VTP as a less invasive method for reinforcing the anterior spinal column, there were some unresolved issues. Firstly, it was observed during the clinical trial that although it was possible to reduce the endplate almost completely with the inflatable bone tamps, a considerable amount of correction was immediately lost after deflation and removal of the balloons. This phenomenon was confirmed by comparing fluoroscopical images obtained during the surgical procedure. Since these images represented the projection of all radiopaque structures in the field of view, including cortical walls, cortical rim and endplate, it was not possible to quantify the actual loss of endplate reduction. The correction loss was probably related to hydrostatic disk pressure, spinal/abdominal muscle tone and/or the presence of large defects under the endplate caused by the inflation of the balloons effectively autografting cancellous bone to the periphery and leading to a decrease in vertical cancellous support [Sato 1999]. Positioning of the balloons under the most impressed part of the endplate was also problematic because of the flexible design of the catheter tips. Recently, unidirectional balloons have been used by other authors to overcome this problem (see chapter 7). To elucidate the biomechanical mechanisms at work during BAER and VTP we quantitatively studied the endplate reduction with a 3D Rotational X-Ray

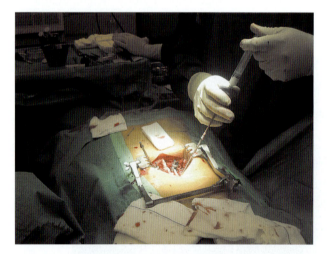

Fig. 67. Intraoperative photograph showing the unilateral technique of injecting cement using the contralateral cannula as overflow channel

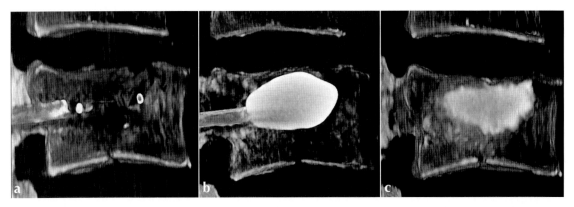

Fig. 68. Chronological series of reconstructed midsagittal 3D rotational X-ray images demonstrating excellent intraoperative imaging of the BAER and VTP procedures

(3DRX) imaging technique in a similar and previously used human cadaveric fracture model [Verlaan 2005]. Using this validated technique it was possible to obtain reconstructions of the spinal specimen in any chosen plane *during* the actual BAER/VTP procedure (Fig. 68a–c). Almost complete endplate reduction was measured after inflation of the balloons [Verlaan, van de Kraats and Oner 2005]. However, a significant amount of correction loss was observed during the interval (typically 30–60 seconds) between deflation of the balloons and injection of cement (see also Fig. 69 for a graphical representation of the correction gained and lost). This loss of endplate reduction will probably be even more pronounced in a clinical setting because of the higher hydrostatic pressure in living hydrated disks and the presence of muscle tone and/or abdominal cavity pressure. Furthermore, the large

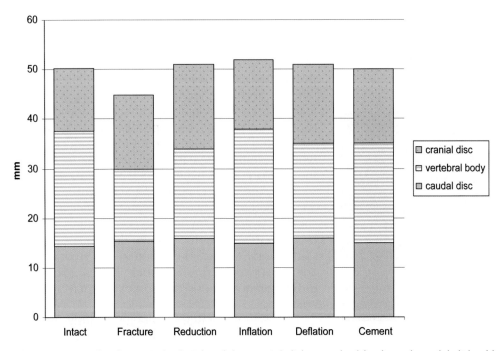

Fig. 69. Bargraphs showing the height of the cranial disk, vertebral body and caudal disk of lumbar specimens during the various phases of the experiment

voids created by the inflatable bone tamps under the fractured endplates may increase the amount of disk intrusion, since structural support of the endplates is obviously decreased at these locations, clearly demonstrated in Fig. 70. Low pressure injection of cement partially restored the endplate reduction by filling the previously created void.

For safety reasons only patients with relatively simple burst fractures demonstrating an intact PLL on preoperative MRI were treated initially. An interesting question would be whether this technique could also safely be used in burst-type fractures with posterior ligamentous complex (PLC) lesions and posterior/anterior longitudinal ligament (PLL/ALL) injuries. Theoretically, an intact PLL and/or ALL could prevent or limit anterior/posterior bone displacement and subsequent cement leakage through the posterior or anterior vertebral body wall respectively. These issues were studied using the 3DRX imaging technique in a modified human cadaveric fracture model in which more severe fractures were created by adding torsion or flexion forces before impact, resulting in PLC, PLL and ALL injuries [Verlaan et al. 2005]. Even when severe ligamentary and bony damage was present, signifying B-type and C-type fractures, it seemed safe to use BAER and VTP in this cadaveric model as we observed no clinically significant increase in anterior/posterior fragment displacement or increase in frequency/amount of cement leakage in comparison to much simpler A-type burst fractures (Fig. 71). Since clinical data on the safety of treating patients with B-type and C-type fractures by BAER and VTP are absent, this technique cannot yet be recommended for routine use.

A combination of external fixation and balloon vertebroplasty for traumatic fractures

The next question would be whether it is really necessary to use adjunctive pedicle screw fixation, which requires considerable soft-tissue dissection, in unstable burst fractures. Pedicle screws are valuable for getting adequate fracture reduction and fixation but, in fracture types with anterior column involvement only, it was hypothesized that these screws might be safely removed after adequate anterior column restoration with BAER and VTP. In his clinical series in the late 1970s, Magerl showed that it was feasible to treat thoracolumbar burst fractures with the external spine fixator (ESF) [Magerl 1984]. Unfortunately, the patients had to carry the ESF for four to five months before healing of the anterior column fracture occurred and subcutaneous infections were numerous. This was the main reason a scaled-down version of the ESF was developed by Dick to be used as a submuscular implant; this device became the original internal fixator [Dick 1985]. With the use of BAER and VTP, it could be feasible to remove the ESP directly after curing of the cement in selected traumatic thoracolumbar fractures (A.3.1; meaning partial burst fractures) with involvement of the anterior column only (Fig. 72a–d). Our first human cadaveric studies in which the ESF was used to reduce and fixate the fracture for the time of the CPC to cure gave promising results but also posed new questions [Verlaan 2004]. Although significant height restoration was feasible with this technique, a considerable and significant loss was observed after applying physiological loads to the augmented spinal segment, raising the question of whether immediate/early ESF removal is a good idea. Before these experimental techniques can be routinely used in clinical practice, further studies are needed to clarify many important clinical issues, such as which AO-type/subtypes fractures to treat or not to treat, what the optimal duration of external spine fixator application is, and whether continuous adjustment of fracture alignment by ESF extension/distraction/dekyphosis during healing may be beneficial.

The new generation of percutaneously inserted pedicle screw constructs may also prove to be an interesting step in reducing collateral soft tissue damage. Although, to the authors' best knowledge,

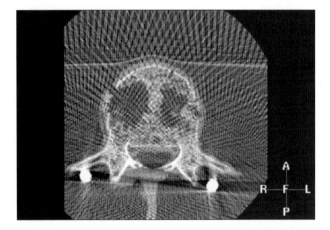

Fig. 70. Reconstructed transverse image of a cadaveric burst fracture after deflation and removal of balloons, demonstrating the resulting large voids in the vertebral body

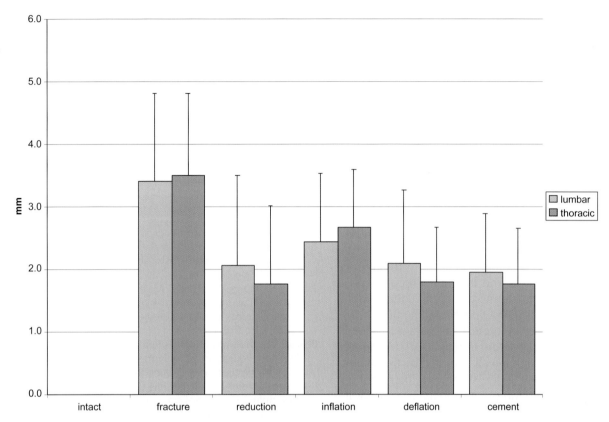

Fig. 71. Bargraph showing posterior bone displacement during instrumented balloon vertebroplasty for both thoracic and lumbar specimens during the various phases of the experiment

no series describing the percutaneous treatment of traumatic fractures have yet been published, some surgeons have used these systems with apparent success [Finiels 2006]. The combination of percutaneously inserted pedicle screw systems in combination with BAER and VTP may provide a less invasive solution for various cases where PLC injury is encountered or suspected.

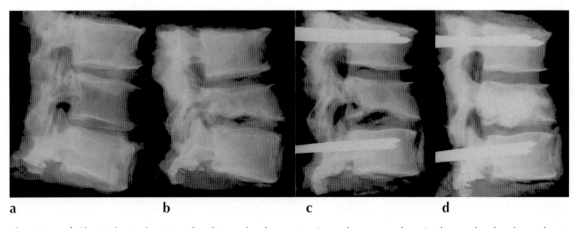

Fig. 72. a–d Chronological series of radiographs demonstrating a human cadaveric thoracolumbar burst fracture treated by external spine fixator, BAER and VTP with calcium phosphate cement

Conclusions

The treatment of thoracolumbar spine fractures has been one of the most contentious subjects in traumatology [Knop 2002; Thomas 2006; Wood 2003]. Difficulties in proper imaging and classification of these injuries have certainly played an important role in the development of many controversies [Oner 1999]. The difficulties in accessing the anterior spinal column and the obvious risks caused by the close proximity and involvement of the dural sac have hampered the application of general trauma surgery principles to the thoracolumbar spine. These factors have led to a higher threshold for surgical treatment of spinal injuries compared with peripheral skeletal injuries. As a result, we have become accustomed to patient-unfriendly treatments such as plaster jackets and long-term recumbency. Moreover, surgeons seem to accept considerable residual deformities following thoracolumbar fractures, something we are typically reluctant to accept in the peripheral skeleton [Shen 2001]. Although spinal deformity may be well tolerated by the majority of trauma patients in the short term, there are no reliable data on the long-term effects of non-physiological biomechanical loading caused by pronounced posttraumatic thoracolumbar kyphosis [Weinstein 1987]. Considering the young age of the average trauma patient and their increased life expectancy, it might not be a good idea to leave these individuals with substantial spinal deformity for the decades to come. However, the present consensus amongst many surgeons, especially in the USA, is to perform surgery only in cases of significant mechanical instability or neurological involvement [Vaccaro 2005]. Better understanding of the basic injury mechanisms and their consequences may enable us to develop operative techniques to repair damage with minimal surgical injury, possibly reducing the long-term discomfort and residual deformity of our patients.

In this chapter a logical series of cadaveric/animal/clinical experiments was presented to assess and discuss the possible benefits and potential risks of using inflatable bone tamps and bone cement in combination with pedicle screw constructs to augment the anterior vertebral column for various traumatic lesions, including dislocated fractures with severe ligamentary instability. The rationale behind these experiments is formed by the hypothesis that anterior spinal column augmentation using a transpedicular approach may decrease the chance of postoperative and long-term kyphosis and the need for secondary, more demanding, anterior or circumferential surgery. BAER and VTP in combination with pedicle screw instrumentation, whether inserted in a classic open approach, inserted percutaneously, or used in combination with an external fixator (the approach largely depending on fracture morphology and injury severity), may play an important role in the development of less invasive surgical methods for treating a large spectrum of thoracolumbar spine fractures.

References

Aebli N, Goss BG, Thorpe P, et al (2006) In vivo temperature profile of intervertebral discs and vertebral endplates during vertebroplasty: an experimental study in sheep. Spine 31: 1674–8

Alanay A, Acaroglu E, Yazici M, et al (2001) The effect of transpedicular intracorporeal grafting in the treatment of thoracolumbar burst fractures on canal remodeling. Eur Spine J 10: 512–6

Belkoff SM, Molloy S (2003) Temperature measurement during polymerization of polymethylmethacrylate cement used for vertebroplasty. Spine 28: 1555–9

Bernhard J, Heini PF, Villiger PM (2003) Asymptomatic diffuse pulmonary embolism caused by acrylic cement: an unusual complication of percutaneous vertebroplasty. Ann Rheum Dis 62: 85–6

Deramond H, Wright NT, Belkoff SM (1999) Temperature elevation caused by bone cement polymerization during vertebroplasty. Bone 25: 17S–21S

Dick W, Kluger P, Magerl F, et al (1985) A new device for internal fixation of thoracolumbar and lumbar spine fractures: the 'fixateur interne'. Paraplegia 23: 225–32

Finiels PJ, Moreau P, Jaume J (2006) The WSH percutaneous spine fixation device. Actual results and future expectations. Neurochirurgie 52: 26–36

Heini PF, Walchli B, Berlemann U (2000) Percutaneous transpedicular vertebroplasty with PMMA: operative technique and early results. A prospective study for the treatment of osteoporotic compression fractures. Eur Spine J 9: 445–50

Knop C, Bastian L, Lange U, et al (2002) Complications in surgical treatment of thoracolumbar injuries. Eur Spine J 11: 214–26

Korovessis P, Baikousis A, Zacharatos S, et al (2006) Combined anterior plus posterior stabilization versus posterior short-segment instrumentation and fusion for midlumbar (L2–L4) burst fractures. Spine 31: 859–68

Magerl F, Aebi M, Gertzbein SD, et al (1994) A comprehensive classification of thoracic and lumbar injuries. Eur Spine J 3: 184–201

Magerl FP (1984) Stabilization of the lower thoracic and lumbar spine with external skeletal fixation. Clin Orthop, pp 125–41

McCormack T, Karaikovic E, Gaines RW (1994) The load sharing classification of spine fractures. Spine 19: 1741–4

Nakano M, Hirano N, Ishihara H, et al (2005) Calcium phosphate cement leakage after percutaneous vertebroplasty for osteoporotic vertebral fractures: risk factor analysis for cement leakage. J Neurosurg Spine 2: 27–33

Nakano M, Hirano N, Matsuura K, et al (2002) Percutaneous transpedicular vertebroplasty with calcium phosphate cement in the treatment of osteoporotic vertebral compression and burst fractures. J Neurosurg 97: 287–93

Oner FC (1999) Thoracolumbar spine fractures: diagnostic and prognostic parameters. Academic Dissertation. University Utrecht

Oner FC, van der Rijt RR, Ramos LM, et al (1998) Changes in the disc space after fractures of the thoracolumbar spine. J Bone Joint Surg Br 80: 833–9

Oner FC, vd Rijt RH, Ramos LM, et al (1999) Correlation of MR images of disc injuries with anatomic sections in experimental thoracolumbar spine fractures. Eur Spine J 8: 194–8

Sato K, Kikuchi S, Yonezawa T (1999) In vivo intradiscal pressure measurement in healthy individuals and in patients with ongoing back problems. Spine 24: 2468–74

Shen WJ, Liu TJ, Shen YS (2001) Nonoperative treatment versus posterior fixation for thoracolumbar junction burst fractures without neurologic deficit. Spine 26: 1038–45

Speth MJ, Oner FC, Kadic MA, et al (1995) Recurrent kyphosis after posterior stabilization of thoracolumbar fractures. 24 cases treated with a Dick internal fixator followed for 1.5–4 years. Acta Orthop Scand 66: 406–10

Thomas KC, Bailey CS, Dvorak MF, et al (2006) Comparison of operative and nonoperative treatment for thoracolumbar burst fractures in patients without neurological deficit: a systematic review. J Neurosurg Spine 4: 351–8

Vaccaro AR, Lehman RA, Jr., Hurlbert RJ, et al (2005) A new classification of thoracolumbar injuries: the importance of injury morphology, the integrity of the posterior ligamentous complex, and neurologic status. Spine 30: 2325–33

Verlaan JJ (2004) Less invasive surgical treatment of traumatic thoracolumbar fractures. Academic Dissertation. University Utrecht

Verlaan JJ, Dhert WJ, Verbout AJ, et al (2005) Balloon vertebroplasty in combination with pedicle screw instrumentation: a novel technique to treat thoracic and lumbar burst fractures. Spine 30: E73–E79

Verlaan JJ, Diekerhof CH, Buskens E, et al (2004) Surgical treatment of traumatic fractures of the thoracic and lumbar spine: a systematic review of the literature on techniques, complications, and outcome. Spine 29: 803–14

Verlaan JJ, Oner FC, Slootweg PJ, et al (2004) Histologic changes after vertebroplasty. J Bone Joint Surg Am 86-A: 1230–8

Verlaan JJ, Oner FC, Verbout AJ, et al (2003) Temperature elevation after vertebroplasty with polymethyl–methacrylate in the goat spine. J Biomed Mater Res 67B: 581–5

Verlaan JJ, van de Kraats EB, Oner FC, et al (2005) Bone displacement and the role of longitudinal ligaments during balloon vertebroplasty in traumatic thoracolumbar fractures. Spine 30: 1832–9

Verlaan JJ, van de Kraats EB, Oner FC, et al (2005) The reduction of endplate fractures during balloon vertebroplasty: a detailed radiological analysis of the treatment of burst fractures using pedicle screws, balloon vertebroplasty, and calcium phosphate cement. Spine 30: 1840–5

Verlaan JJ, van de Kraats EB, van Walsum T, et al (2005) Three-dimensional rotational X-ray imaging for spine surgery: a quantitative validation study comparing reconstructed images with corresponding anatomical sections. Spine 30: 556–61

Verlaan JJ, van Helden WH, Oner FC, et al (2002) Balloon vertebroplasty with calcium phosphate cement augmentation for direct restoration of traumatic thoracolumbar vertebral fractures. Spine 27: 543–8

Weinstein JN, Collalto P, Lehmann TR (1987) Long-term follow-up of nonoperatively treated thoracolumbar spine fractures. J Orthop Trauma 1: 152–9

Wood K, Butterman G, Mehbod A, et al (2003) Operative compared with nonoperative treatment of a thoracolumbar burst fracture without neurological deficit. A prospective, randomized study. J Bone Joint Surg Am 85-A: 773–81

Percutaneous kyphoplasty in traumatic fractures

G. Maestretti, S. Krajinovic, and P. Otten

Terminology

Kyphoplasty: A method of percutaneous restoration of the shape of vertebral bodies with the aim of correction of a traumatic kyphotic deformity
IBT: Inflatable bone tamp
VAS: Visual analog scale
CPC: Calcium phosphate cement
PMMA: Polymethyl methacrylate
VCF: Vertebral compression fracture

Introduction

Ninety percent of all traumatic spinal fractures occur in the thoracolumbar region and 66% of these are type A (A1 35%, A2 3.5%, A3 27.5%) compression fractures mainly involving the vertebral body (VB) [Magerl et al. 1994]. The posterior column presents only minor injuries, if at all. The height of the VB is reduced, but the posterior ligamentous complex is intact. Translation in the sagittal plane does not occur. Typical axial compression with or without flexion causes this type of injury. The incidence of neurological injuries increases to approximately 32% in burst fractures of type A3 (Fig. 73) [Liebermann et al. 2001]. Although this is a very common fracture, there is no consensus on standard treatment. Various opinions have been expressed on the best appropriate treatment for those fractures without neurological deficit and it remains a subject of controversy [Ooms et al. 2003a; Shen et al. 2001]. Internal fixation offers immediate stability and the possibility of correcting a major deformity, if necessary even with decompression of neurological structures. Non-operative care with a brace or body cast offers the same possibility of stability, although with lesser correction of deformity [Mainard et al. 2003; Ooms et al. 2003a, b]. In Wood et al. [2003] published long-term results of a randomized study comparing conservative treatment with the surgical instrumented technique and did not find any advantage for surgery [Wood et al. 2003].

Failed stability after pedicle screw fixation and especially after removal of instrumentation or after conservative management is possibly due to lesions of the disc and later to disc degeneration with decreased anterior column support [Oner et al. 1998; Mainard et al. 2003]. Restoration of vertebral height and preservation of the endplate may prevent the secondary risk of kyphotic deformation and also reduce the risk of chronic pain.

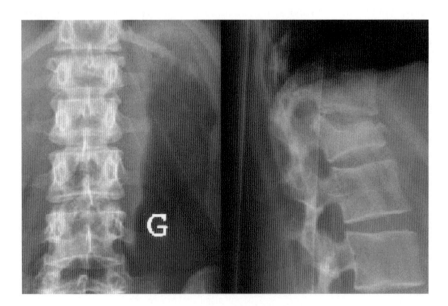

Fig. 73. Example of a type A3.2 fracture of the L1 vertebra

Kyphoplasty was developed for the treatment of painful osteoporotic compression fractures and for VB height restoration and cement augmentation, and the technique has shown a lower complication rate than vertebroplasty [Eck et al. 2007; Fujikawa et al. 1995; Kopylov et al. 1996].

The introduction of CPCs with better biocompatibility [Brown and Chow 1983; Chow et al. 1998; Driessens et al. 1993, 2002; Fernandez et al. 1998; Frankenburg et al. 1998; Hutton et al. 2000; Khairoun et al. 1997, 1998; Tomita et al. 2003] than PMMA and with enough resistance under compression [Tomita et al. 2003] has enabled, in association with kyphoplasty, new treatment in some type A fractures in young patients.

History of kyphoplasty

Kyphoplasty was developed independently of vertebroplasty in the 1980s by an orthopedic surgeon looking for a minimally invasive surgical procedure for dealing with the pain and deformity of vertebral compression fractures (VCFs) and which would follow orthopedic principles: anatomy restoration and solid fixation while minimizing tissue disruption.

The first balloon kyphoplasty procedure for osteoporotic VCF was performed by Dr. M. Reiley in Berkeley California in 1998. The CE mark was obtained in February 2000.

In standard kyphoplasty procedure, an inflatable bone tamp (IBT) or balloon is used to restore the height of the vertebral body and correct the spinal deformities before cementation.

The technique shares similarities with vertebroplasty only in the use of percutaneous intrabody cannulae for cement injection; however, kyphoplasty has a number of potential advantages, such as a lower risk of cement extravazation and the potential for better restoration of vertebral height.

The idea of using this technique to treat traumatic fractures in young patients appeared in three European groups independently of each other. The first standalone kyphoplasty procedure with a CPC for traumatic fractures was performed in Belgium by Prof. P. Vanderschot in July 2002. At the same time two other groups started using the same technique: in Switzerland Dr. G. Maestretti and Dr. P. Otten, and in Germany Dr. H. Hillmeier.

The first advisory team meeting, regrouping the Kyphon Trauma Group (Dr. Ortner Austria; Dr. Francanella, Italy; Prof. Dr. Vanderschot, Belgium; Dr. Maestretti, Switzerland; Dr. Hillmeier, Germany),

was held in Belgium in March 2003 with the aim of better defining the indications and laying the foundations for standardization of this technique.

Advantages of percutaneous kyphoplasty

This minimally invasive technique offers the advantage of a lower risk of morbidity, thus allowing a quicker return to daily activities, work and sports. The immediate disappearance of pain with minimal operative risks and guaranteed biomechanical stability of the fractured vertebra offer advantages over the standard treatment.

As blood loss is minimal, kyphoplasty could be a first choice technique in polytraumatized patients needing short-term stabilization of the spine, thus improving nursing in ICU without any risk of secondary lesions.

The technique of kyphoplasty enables normal mobilization after six hours, depending on residual pain, without a brace. Patients can be discharged from the hospital the same day that the operation took place.

Disadvantages of percutaneous kyphoplasty

This technique is an operation and is preferably performed under general anesthesia even though it is minimally invasive; it also necessitates extensive use of fluoroscopy.

The technique uses the same approach as a kyphoplasty in osteoporotic fractures but the application of the CPC is more difficult, mainly because of the short crystallization time, which makes it difficult to apply the cement and necessitates a long learning curve.

The initial cost is high, because of the price of IBTs, but we believe this cost is balanced out by the short hospitalization and a faster return to work.

Indications for percutaneous kyphoplasty

The Kyphon trauma group reached consensus on the following indications: traumatic fractures of types A1 and A3.1, involving vertebral bodies from Th5 to L5, without any neurological deficit, with at least 15° of VB deformity (angle inferior versus superior plate) in monotrauma lesion or 10° in polytraumatized patients or with multilevel fractures. In type A2 fractures with a split less than 2 mm and in A3.2 fractures greater experience with standalone traumatic kyphoplasty is necessary and in most cases PMMA cementation is advised. Kyphoplasty may be considered in types A3.3, B and C fractures associated with posterior instrumentation.

Contraindications

Contraindications are given for fractures at high thoracic level above Th5, cervical fractures, type A2 fractures with a split larger than 2 mm, fracture types A3.3, B and C in standalone kyphoplasty. Pathological fractures and fractures older than three weeks are not treated with this technique. Pregnancy, infection and any contraindication for general anesthesia also exclude treatment by kyphoplasty.

Surgical technique

Kyphoplasty technique in traumatic fractures

Preoperative CT evaluation of the fracture line is mandatory in traumatic fractures. An ideal planification of the placement (in two planes) of the cannulae and the IBT is necessary for VB reconstruction (Figs. 74 and 75).

In order to facilitate spontaneous reduction of the fracture, the patient is in prone position with lordosis. Sometimes this positioning of the patient already results in reduction of eventually present posterior fragments. A fluoroscopic C-Arm is set for AP and lateral images. Just as in standard balloon kyphoplasty (Kyphon), an inflatable bone tamp (IBT or balloon) is used to restore the VB height and correct the spinal deformities and the VB endplate before cementation. Nevertheless, there are some main differences from the standard kyphoplasty for osteoporosis: after the correct identification of the involved level, Yamshidi cannulae are placed under fluoroscopy in a trajectory 2 mm inferior and parallel to the fracture line, ideally into it, via either a trans- or an extrapedicular route, taking care to stay a few millimeters under the fractured endplate (Figs. 76 and 77). The planning of the procedure and trajectory of the cannulae, also the choice of route, depends on the fracture location and the anatomy as seen on the pre-operative CT scan (Figs. 74 and 75).

The choice of size and type of IBT depends on the size of the VB, the amount of reduction needed and the type of fracture. For example, in an A3.1 fracture at the Th10 level a 4-cc balloon is preferred and is placed in the anterior third portion of the vertebra to minimize the risk of posterior fragment displacement into the canal. The two IBTs, filled with radio-opaque medium, are simultaneously inflated up to 50 psi and then progressively inflated by 0.5 ml under lateral fluoroscopy guidance (Figs. 78 and 79).

In young patients with acute fractures and good bone quality, high pressures of 300 psi are quickly obtained, with a low-volume IBT. With optimal po-

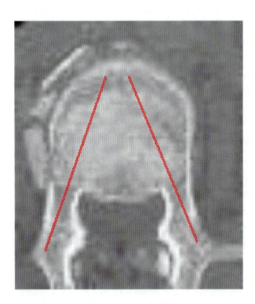

Fig. 74. Axial planning, ideal trajectory to obtain "kissing balloons"

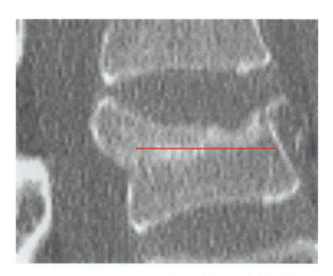

Fig. 75. Sagittal planning, 2 mm inferior to the fracture line

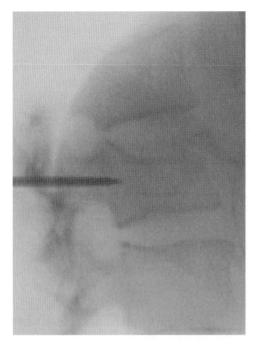

Fig. 76. Lateral view of the Yamshidi cannula which is introduced transpedicularly

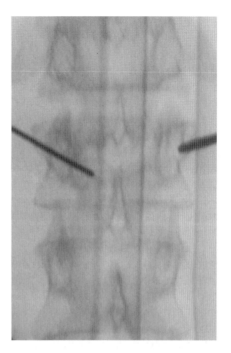

Fig. 77. AP view (left-hand side: guide pin, right-hand side: Yamshidi cannula)

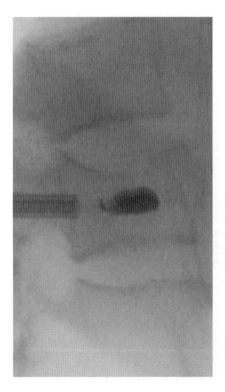

Fig. 78. Filling of the balloons with radio-opaque medium under lateral fluoroscopic guidance

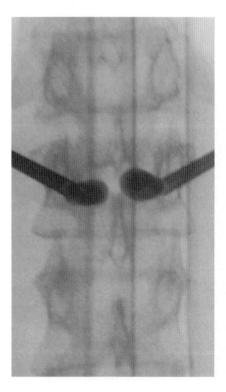

Fig. 79. AP view of the balloon position

sition of the balloons and a little bit of perseverance, progressive displacement of the trabeculae and correction of the fracture are obtained and the initial high pressure should decrease while the balloons reduce the fracture and expand themselves. Operative time is proportional to the type and age of the fracture and the degree of VB kyphosis, and may take more than 1 h. To avoid rupture of the balloons, maximal pressure of 430 psi and a respective total volume must not be exceeded.

When satisfactory reduction of the fracture has been obtained, both IBTs are removed and the bone cavity created by the IBT is filled with cement. In case of loss of correction after removal of the balloons, a two-time cementation is used: one balloon is refilled without contrast agent and replaced in the VB on the side of the greatest deformity. Thus, the endplate is restored again and the other half of the VB can be cemented first; after removal of the balloon the second half is cemented. Calcibon™ (Biomet Merck) is kept in a refrigerator and in order to delay the crystallization time it is mixed just before use. With the new CPC KyphOs™ this step is not necessary as the handling and setting times are longer. Mixing is always performed by pouring the liquid first then adding the powder and stirring for 60 s to obtain a viscous consistency. Kyphon 1.5 cc bone fillers are pre-filled quickly. The distal end is obtruded with bone wax to protect the cement from early contact with blood, as blood also increases the crystallization of Calcibon™. Cementation of the VB with a CPC starts in the anterior part and proceeds posteriorly, under constant lateral fluoroscopy (Figs. 80 and 81), paying special attention to posterior fragments in type A3 fractures. This very short phase takes approximately 3 minutes but is difficult to perform and needs extensive experience with conventional PMMA cement (Figs. 84 and 85) to achieve full cementation of the VB. After crystallization the cannulae are removed, a final fluoroscopy check is performed and the skin is sutured.

Calcium phosphate cement

CPCs consist of a powder containing one or more solid compounds of calcium and/or phosphate salts and a cement liquid that can be water or an aqueous solution [Bai et al. 1999]. If the powder and the liquid are mixed in an appropriate ratio, they form a paste that at room or body temperature sets by entanglement of the crystals precipitated within the paste [Tomita et al. 2003; Verlaan et al. 2002]. The

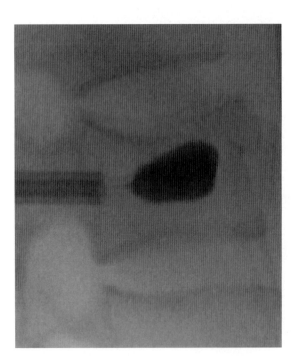

Fig. 80. Progressive inflation of the balloons

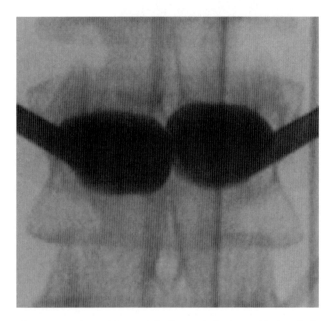

Fig. 81. End position of balloon inflation ("kissing balloons")

Percutaneous kyphoplasty in traumatic fractures

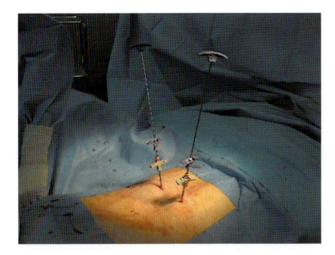

Fig. 82. Balloons are yet removed, insertion of the cement filling cannulae on both sides

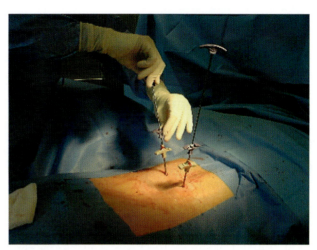

Fig. 83. Cement application

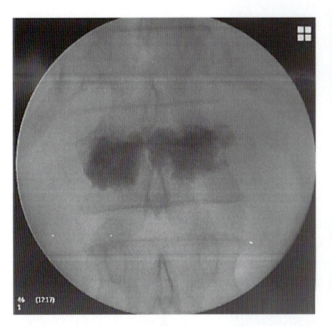

Fig. 84. Result with PMMA cement in AP view

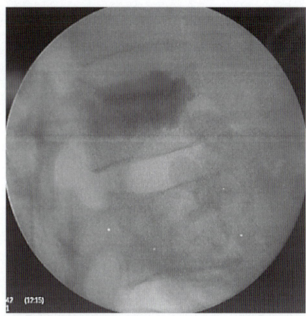

Fig. 85. Result with PMMA cement in lateral view

material can be shaped for several minutes and is, depending on the liquid-to-powder (L/P) ratio, injectable via a syringe [Brown and Chow 1983; Chow et al. 1998]. One of the most important characteristics of CPC is its ability to be osteoconductive and degradable [Driessens et al. 1993, 2000; Khairoun et al. 1997, 1998].

Although numerous reports have been published on in vitro and in vivo CPC investigations, there are still some problems to overcome [Wolke et al. 1999]. These mainly involve the setting time and the degradation rate of the cement in vivo, whereas the compressive strength reached after setting has been much improved [Frankenburg et al. 1998; Hillmeier et al. 2004]. Calcibon™ has been available for clinical use since June 2002 and for vertebral augmentation since 2006. Mixing the powder with a liquid (disodium hydrogen phosphate) at an L/P ratio of 0.35 produces a paste with a cohesion time of 1 min, initial setting time of 3 min and final setting time of 7.5 min at 37°C without exothermic reaction. A compressive strength of 30 MPa is reached at 6 h and 60 MPa at 3 days [Ooms et al. 2000; Wenz et al. 2000]. A biologic improved osteotransduction capacity after 6 months without cellular toxicity or mutation has been confirmed in animal studies [Ooms et al. 2002a, b; Ooms et al. 2003a, b; Verlaan et al. 2002].

Calcibon™ is composed of 61% α-tricalcium phosphate (TCP), 26% calcium hydrogen phosphate,

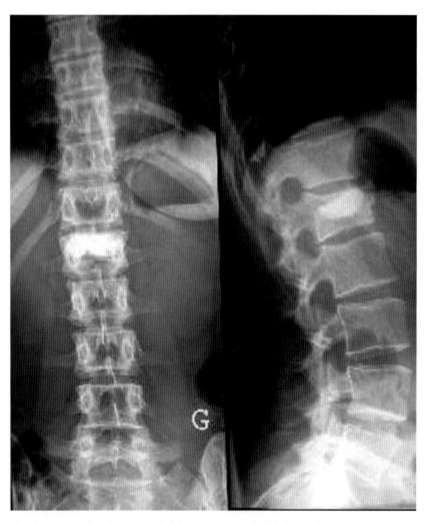

Fig. 86. Example of a type A3.2 fracture treated with CPC, 1 year post-operatively (same patient as in Fig. 72)

10% calcium carbonate and 3% hydroxyapatite. The cement paste hardens as a CDHA trough hydrolysis of the α-TCP:

3 Ca$_3$(PO$_4$)$_2$ + H$_2$O → Ca$_9$(HPO$_4$)(PO$_4$)$_5$OH

Calcibon™ complies with the stated requirements when mixed at L/P ratios of 0.30–0.40 and is injectable via a syringe at L/P ratios of 0.33–0.40.

Cell culture studies using fibroblast and human bone marrow osteoprogenitor cells have shown that the material is not cytotoxic and that it stimulates differentiation of osteoblasts. Osteoclast response to the cement in tissue culture showed that the material was reabsorbed by osteoclasts.

The newer material, KyphOs™ shows optimal characteristics at an L/P ratio of 0.4. It consists of an α-TCP 77.4%, magnesium phosphate 14.3%, magnesium hydrogen phosphate 4.7% and strontium carbonate 3.6%. A compressive strength of 6.1 MPa is reached at 20 min after mixing, 120 MPa after 120 min and 105 MPa at 24 hours [Schwardt et al. 2006].

Postoperative care

Depending on the patient's residual pain, mobilization can start from the 6th postoperative hour after cementation with Calcibon™ or KyphOs. After the use of PMMA, mobilization can begin at 3 hours

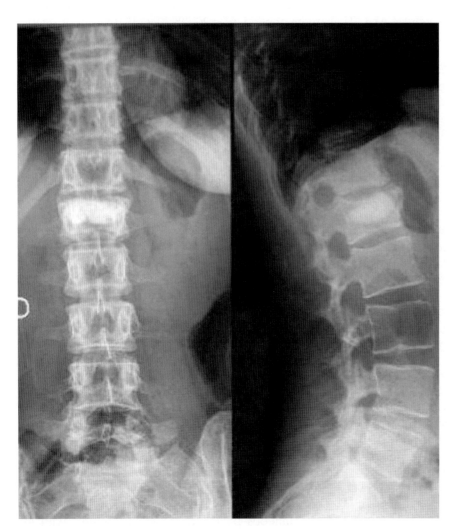

Fig. 87. Example of a type A3.2 fracture treated with CPC, 2 years post-operatively (same patient as in Figs. 73 and following)

postoperatively. We advise patients not to lift any load and to avoid physical effort for a period of two weeks.

Gentle decontracting massages are prescribed, with isometric muscular reinforcement. Standard advice for good back posture is given by a physiotherapist. After two weeks the patient may return to work and take part in sport; any delays are due to residual post-traumatic muscle contraction.

Results of our study

Between August 2002 and August 2003, 28 patients (10 female and 18 male) under the mean age of 38 (17–64) were treated for a total of 33 acute traumatic type A vertebral fractures without neurology. The follow-up with a mean of 30 months was 100%. Six patients had additional fractures. The affected levels were T11 (4), T12 (4), L1 (6), L2 (9), L3 (7), L4 (2) and L5 (1). The types of fractures were 3 A1.1, 21 A1.2, 7 A3.1 and 2 A3.2 and the operation was performed at a mean of 3.4 (1–21) days after injury. The mean surgery time was 60 (35–90) min. The mean final pressure of the IBT was 233 (180–400) psi and in all cases substantial reduction of fractured endplate was achieved. The mean volume of Calcibon injected was 6.8 (4.5–9) ml. The blood loss was insignificant. No adverse hemodynamic events were detected per-operatively. The mean initial pre-operative vertebral kyphosis, measured in supine position, was 17° (0–24°); the mean per-operative reduction obtained was 5° (0–9°). We noticed a loss of correction from a mean of 6° (0–11°) in the standing X-rays at 24 h to a mean of 9° (0–17°) at the last follow-up (P = 0.001). The mean segmental kyphosis in supine position was 3° (–36° to +26°) pre-operatively, –6° (–28° to +20°) per-operatively, –1° (–38° to +22°) post-operatively at 24 h (standing X-rays), and –1° (–32° to +28°) at the last follow-up (P = 0.071). The height restoration (Beck Index) was 0.70 (0.50–0.90) pre-operatively, corrected to 0.90 (0.81–1) per-operatively, 0.87 (0.81–1) post-operatively at 24 h, and 0.84 (0.76–1) at the last follow-up (P = 0.002). The loss of correction was not significantly correlated with the clinical outcome. The VAS decreased over time from a pre-operative mean of 8.7 (7–10), to 3.1 (0–5) at 7 days and 1 (0–4) at the last follow-up (P = 0.001).

The Roland–Morris disability score improved similarly during the follow-up from a mean of 3 (0–12) at 7 days to 2 (0–9) at the last follow-up (7 days post-operatively and at 2 years, P = 0.004).

Only the post-operative Roland-Morris data are reported because most of the patients are young and presented a normal score before the accident. All patients with isolated vertebral fractures (N = 22) recovered uneventfully without neurological deficit and were discharged within 48 h and returned to the same work within 3 months with the same working ability as before the accident. No long-term clinical complications were detected at the last follow-up. In the majority of cases the cement was not completely substituted at the last follow-up. On CT scan we found partial cement resorption starting after 6 months without visible bone formation. In the biopsy at 12 months we found an image (Fig. 88) showing normal fracture healing and new bone formation without signs of inflammation or necrosis. High variability of cement resorption was confirmed by CT measurement (24 h, 1 year). The mean resorption, in reference to the initial volume of cement applied, was 20.3% (0.3–35.3%) and is related to the individual biological resorption process. We found no correlation between the kind of fracture, the clinical outcome and the amount of resorption of the cement. The new bone formation was not measurable. In the patients with A1.1 and A1.2 fractures we did not see any segmental decompensation at the last follow-up. In the patients with A3.1 and A3.2 fractures (nine cases) we obtained spontaneous fusion in the worst case (1/9) or partial loss of correction (4/9); in the other cases we did not notice decompensation of the disc (4/9) [21].

Complications

At July 2007 we had treated a total of 120 patients with this technique, not only those in the cited study. We have had to re-operate in a total of two cases: one type B and one A3.3 fracture that showed VB kyphosis in the immediate postoperative X-ray. We noticed some technical operative complications: two anterior wall perforations by cannulae and six cement leakages. Those leakages are defined as any cement contact in the disc space that can be observed on the post-operative radiographs or on the CT scan. In one case we observed a small leakage in the lateral portion of the spinal canal without clinical significance. Such leakages certainly occur through fracture lines, since we never noticed any leakage in veins or any pulmonary embolism.

Long-term results demonstrated a 30% risk of spontaneous balanced fusion in fractures with involved disc lesions without clinical relevance.

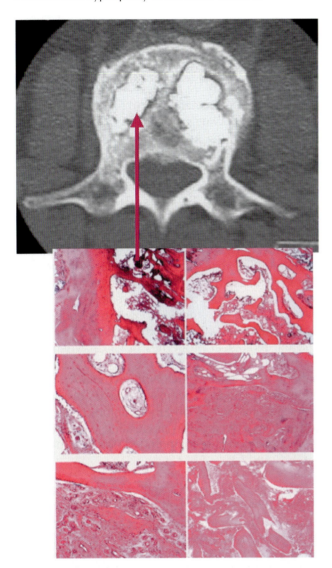

Fig. 88. Biopsy site and histological result 1 year post-operatively showing complete integration of the CPC with new bone formation

Critical evaluation

The standard treatment for thoracolumbar vertebral type A fractures is still debated. Conservative treatment does not restore spinal balance and, because of the loss of anterior height, this may lead to acceleration of disc degeneration and loss of anterior support.

Open surgical therapy with instrumentation carries definite risks and is destructive to muscles, but it helps to restore vertebral height, thus preventing the long-term chronic pain sometimes seen in post-traumatic kyphotic deformations. Kyphoplasty is a new technique in the treatment of osteoporotic fractures resistant to conservative therapy and appears in some ways to be superior to vertebroplasty, as the risk of complications such as cement leakage and venous embolism is reduced, and also a greater risk of new fracture [Eck et al. 2007]. Nevertheless, the databanks of scientific publications offer poor results for searches on the use of kyphoplasty in traumatic fractures: a couple of case reports present the still limited knowledge and/or use of this technique for this indication.

In our study [Maestretti et al. 2007] we demonstrated the feasibility and safety of this new, less invasive technique for reduction and direct stabilization of the anterior column after acute type A VB fractures. Advantages of this minimally invasive technique are an almost immediate return to daily activities, disappearance of pain, minimal operative risks and maintenance of stability. In addition, blood loss is minimal and this could be a first-choice technique in polytraumatized patients needing rapid stabilization of the spine, thus improving nursing in the intensive care unit. This technique enables normal mobilization after 6 h, depending on residual muscular pain, without any brace. The patients can be discharged home the same day. In comparison with conservative treatment with a brace, kyphoplasty patients do not have to bear so much inconvenience and they have a better reduction of the fracture and better control of pain under load. Compared with standard surgery, this technique offers a reduced risk of morbidity [Müller et al. 1999; Oner et al. 1998; Resch et al. 2000; Trivedi 2002]. The immediate stability leads to rapid reduction of pain, allowing a quicker return to work and sports activity. Our study shows that treatment of type A thoracolumbar fractures with kyphoplasty compares well with the standard treatments [Shen et al. 2001; Wood et al. 2003]. We obtain the benefit of a minimally invasive percutaneous technique and, with regard to the final kyphosis, achieve the same radiological results as in classic surgical technique, but with better clinical outcomes [Bai et al. 1999; Tomita et al. 2003; Verlaan et al. 2002]. Comparable results have been obtained in a recently published study by Hillmeier et al. [2004] comparing kyphoplasty with PMMA or CPC in osteoporotic and traumatic fractures either as a standalone technique or with associated posterior fixation. Nevertheless, although it is minimally invasive, the technique of kyphoplasty is an operation necessitating general anesthesia and extensive use of fluoroscopy. The technique uses the same approach as kyphoplasty in osteoporotic fracture but the application of the CPC is more demanding, mainly because of the short crystallization time and the difficulty of application, which necessitates a long learning curve. Cement cracks and lacunas around the cement were observed in all CT scans at 1 year, but without any impact on the clinical findings.

Despite histological examinations, we found no reasonable explanation for the lacunas. We hypothesize that they correspond to a normal early stage of cement substitution with bone. If the cement crack appears in the first week it will increase the risk of acute kyphotic decompensation. This can be explained by a variety of combined factors: on the one hand the severe injury of an A3 fracture leads to significant endplate damage or associated disc ruptures and thence to disturbed pathways of disc nutrition; on the other hand incorrect application of cement could also be the cause of disturbed crystal formation and consequent change in the intrinsic properties of the cement.

In cases of severe A3.1, A3.2 and A3.3 fractures we do not recommend the use of CPC and kyphoplasty in a standalone fashion, because of the low shearing stability resulting from the intrinsic characteristic of this biological cement. In such cases, we suggest the use of PMMA to achieve a better shearing stability. Further development of cements is necessary to improve handling, intrinsic capacity for shearing resistance and also the biological osteotransduction. In an animal study comparing the histological reaction to CPC or PMMA in a VB and in contact with the disc, Verlaan et al. [2004] concluded that vertebroplasty can be performed with both of these cements without increased risk of disc or endplate degeneration, even when endplate discontinuity is present. Burst fractures of type A3 and some type A2 are accompanied with fractures of the endplate and lesions of the disc. The endplate is the main nutritional pathway to the disc and therefore disturbance of the endplate could lead to impairment of vascularization and transport of nutrients. Many studies have demonstrated the progressive degeneration and poor regenerative capacity of the disc once a part of the annulus has been damaged [Adams et al. 2000; Hadjipavlou et al. 1999; Hutton et al. 2000]. In an MRI study, Oner et al. [1998, 1999] found that fracture of the endplate resulted in redistribution of disc material through the endplate in the VB but did not lead to disc de-

generation. We found no significant loss of segmental correction after two years, neither in type A1 fractures (P = 0.107) nor in A3 fractures (P = 0.231). In our opinion, restoration of the endplate to preserve the mobility of associated segments could maintain the vascularization and the pump nutrition in the disc, allowing it to heal, but only in young patients and in the lower lumbar level. Only long-term follow-up will confirm this hypothesis.

The initial cost of balloon kyphoplasty is high because of the price of IBTs, but the cost benefit could be balanced by the shorter hospitalization and shorter period of inactivity. The high rate of early return to normal daily activities and work is especially beneficial. Our two-year results of the study and five years of experience seem to indicate that kyphoplasty and cementation with CPC can be used as a potential alternative treatment for acute thoracolumbar fractures. Long-term studies are needed to assess the maintenance of disc height and the biological properties of CPC. When using Calcibon™ or KyphOS™ we recommend standalone balloon kyphoplasty only in type A1 and A3.1 acute fractures in young patients (< 40 years of age). For older patients and in unstable fracture patterns the use of PMMA cement in association with posterior instrumentation is recommended (fractures of types A3.3, B and C).

References

Adams MA, et al (2000) Mechanical initiation of intervertebral disc degeneration. Spine 25: 1625–1636

Bai B, et al (1999) The use of an injectable, biodegradable calcium phosphate bone substitute for the prophylactic augmentation of osteoporotic vertebrae and the management of vertebral compression fractures. Spine 24: 1521–1526

Brown WE, Chow LC (1983) A new calcium phosphate setting cement. J Dent Res 2: 62

Chow LC, et al (1998) Calcium phosphate cements. Cements Res Prog, pp 215–238

Daniaux H (1986) Transpedicular repositioning and spongioplasty in fractures of the vertebral bodies of the lower thoracic and lumbar spine. Unfallchirurg 89(5): 197–213

Driessens FC, et al (1993) Formulation and setting times of some calcium orthophosphate cements: a pilot study. J Mater Sci Mater Med 4: 503–508

Driessens FC, Boltong MG, Wenz R (2000) Calcium phosphate bone cements: state of the art 2000. 12th Conference of the European Society of Biomechanics, Dublin, Ireland

Driessens FC, et al (2002) Comparative study of some experimental or commercial calcium phosphate bone cements. Bioceramics, vol 11. Proceedings of the 11th International Symposium on Ceramics in Medicine, pp 231–233

Eck JC, et al (2007) Comparison of vertebroplasty and balloon kyphoplasty for treatment of vertebral compression fractures: a meta-analysis of the literature. Review article. Spine (in press) Epub ahead of print

Fernandez E, Gil FJ, Best SM, Ginebra MP, Driessens FC, Planell JA (1998) Improvement of the mechanical properties of new calcium phosphate bone cements in the $CaHPO_4$-alpha-$Ca_3(PO_4)_2$ system: compressive strength and microstructural development. J Biomed Mater Res 41: 560–567

Frankenburg EP, et al (1998) Biomechanical and histological evaluation of calcium phosphate cement. J Bone Joint Surg Am 80(8): 1112–1124

Fujikawa K, et al (1995) Histopathological reaction of calcium phosphate cement in periodontal bone defect. Dent Mater J 14: 45–57

Garfin SR, et al (2001) New technologies in spine: kyphoplasty and vertebroplasty for the treatment of painful osteoporotic compression fractures. Spine 26(14): 1511–1515

Hadjipavlou AG, et al (1999) Pathomechanics and clinical relevance of disc degeneration and annular tear: a point-of-view review. Am J Orthop 28: 561–571

Hillmeier J, et al (2004) Augmentation von Wirbelkörperfrakturen mit einem neuen Calciumphosphate-Zement nach Ballon-Kyphoplastie. Orthopäde 33: 31–39

Hutton WC, et al (2000) Does long-term compressive loading on the intervertebral disc cause degeneration? Spine 25: 2993–3004

Khairoun I, Boltong MG, Driessens FC, Planell JA (1997) Effect of calcium carbonate on clinical compliance of apatitic calcium phosphate bone cement. J Biomed Mater Res 38(4): 356–360

Khairoun I, et al (1998) Some factors controlling the injectability of calcium phosphate bone cement. J Mater Sci Mater Med 9: 425–428

Kopylov P, et al (1996) Injectable calcium phosphate in the treatment of distal radial fractures. J Hand Surg Br 21: 768–771

Liebermann I, et al (2001) Initial outcome and efficacy of kyphoplasty in the treatment of painful osteoporotic vertebral compression fractures. Spine 26(14): 1631–1638

Maestretti, et al (2007) Prospective study of standalone balloon kyphoplasty with calcium phosphate cement augmentation in traumatic fractures. Eur Spine J 16(5) : 601–10

Magerl F, et al (1994) A comprehensive classification of thoracic and lumbar injuries. Eur Spine J 3: 184–201

Mainard D, et al (2003) Les substituts osseux en 2003. Romillat, Paris

Müller U, et al (1999) Treatment of thoracolumbar burst fractures without neurological deficit by indirect reduction and posterior instrumentation: bisegmental stabilization with monosegmental fusion. Eur Spine J 8: 284–289

Oner FC, et al (1998) Changes in the disc space after fractures of the thoracolumbar spine. J Bone Joint Surg Br 80: 833–839

Oner FC, et al (1999) MRI findings of thoracolumbar spine fractures: a categorisation based on MRI examination of 100 fractures. Skeletal Radiol 28: 433–443

Ooms EM, Wolke JCG, Jansen JA (2000) Evaluation of a high strength calcium phosphate bone cement. 6th World Biomaterials Congress, Hawaii

Ooms EM, Wolke JGC, van der Waerden JPCM, Jansen JA (2002a) Trabecular bone response to injectable calcium phosphate (Ca-P) cement. J Biomed Mater Res 61: 9–18

Ooms E, et al (2002b) Trabecular bone response to injectable calcium phosphate (Ca-P) cement. Wiley, New York (www.interscience.wiley.com)

Ooms EM, Egglezos EA, Wolke JGC, Jansen JA (2003a) Soft-tissue response to injectable calcium phosphate cements. Biomaterials 24: 749–757

Ooms EM, Wolke JCG, van de Heuvel MT, Jeschke B, Jansen JA (2003b) Histological evaluation of the bone response to calcium phosphate cement implanted in cortical bone. Biomaterials 24: 989–1000

Resch H, et al (2000) Operative vs. konservative Behandlung von Frakturen des thorakolumbalen Übergangs. Unfallchirurg 103: 281–288

Schwardt J, et al (2006) KyphOs™ FS Calcium phosphate for balloon kyphoplasty: verification of compressive strength and instructions for use. European Cells and Materials 11 [Suppl 1]: 28

Shen WJ, et al (2001) Nonoperative treatment versus posterior fixation for thoracolumbar junction burst fractures without neurologic deficit. Spine 26(9): 1038–1045

Tomita S, et al (2003) Biomechanical evaluation of kyphoplasty and vertebroplasty with calcium phosphate cement in a simulated osteoporotic compression fracture. J Orthop Sci 8: 192–197

36. Trivedi JM (2002) Spinal trauma: therapy options and outcomes. Eur J Radiol 42: 127–134

Verlaan JJ, et al (2002) Balloon vertebroplasty with calcium phosphate cement augmentation for direct restoration of traumatic thoracolumbar vertebral fracture. Spine 27(5): 543–548

Verlaan JJ, et al (2004) Histological changes after vertebroplasty. J Bone Joint Surg 86: 1230–1238

Wenz R, Boltong MG, Driessens FC (2000) Calcium phosphate bone cements: state of the art 1999. 6th World Biomaterials Congress, Hawaii

Wolke JGC, Wenz R, Ooms EM, Boltong MG, Driessens FC, Jansen JA (1999) Physiochemical properties, composition and in vivo resorption behaviour of a high strength calcium phosphate cement. Concepts and clinical applications on ionic cements. 15th European Conference on Biomaterials, Arcachon, Bordeaux, France

Wood K, et al (2003) Operative compared with non-operative treatment of a thoracolumbar burst fracture without neurological deficit. J Bone J Surg 85(5): 773–781

Chapter 11

Alternative methods to kyphoplasty: vertebroplasty – lordoplasty

P. F. Heini and R. Orler

Percutaneous cement augmentation (vertebroplasty) was used for the first time in the 1980s, primarily for treatment of vertebral hemangioma [Galibert 1987]. It was only in the middle of the 1990s that it was used for treatment of metastases and increasingly for osteoporotic fractures of the spine [Cotten 1996; Weill 1996; Jensen 1997; Cortet 1999; Heini 2000]. In the meantime, this method has become established for treatment of painful osteoporotic fractures and for tumorous osteolysis of the spine. The clinical success rate is very high, with rapid pain relief in 70–90% of treated patients [Legroux-Gerot 2004; Zoarski 2002; Peh 2002; Barr 2000].

Patient evaluation

The case history plays a central role in the assessment of patients with a possible osteoporotic fracture. Radiological evaluation of the painful section of spine should be carried out in patients complaining of pain that occurred spontaneously or after a traumatic event. The initial symptoms after a fracture are quite uniform in presentation, with considerable cingulate pain. Slowly subsiding pain is an indication of increasing solidification of the broken vertebra; continual strong pain indicates a continuing sintering process. These patients should be closely monitored with radiology. Patients who complain of mechanical backache over weeks and months, especially when changing from a lying into a sitting position, possibly suffer from "pseudoarthrosis". This instability can be diagnosed by comparing x-rays taken in a standing and in a lying position. Patients with a neurologic deficit (motor deficit, ataxia, radicular pain, claudication symptoms) should be diagnosed by means of MRI, CT or myelogram.

The clinical examination often shows a painful response to percussion in the fractured area. The pain is, however, frequently located deeper than the actual fracture. The sagittal balance of the spine is often disturbed in patients with high-grade osteoporosis and multiple fractures. All patients should undergo neurological assessment.

In addition to clarifying the local findings, the personal case history (general condition, risk factors and medication) should be reviewed.

Radiological evaluation

The preferred examination method at initial presentation of an osteoporotic vertebral fracture is a conventional radiograph of the corresponding section of spine in two planes; this should be done with the patient in a standing position if possible.

MRI examination is suited best for determining the age of the fracture. Edema in the vertebral body indicates persisting activity. Scintigraphy of the skeleton can also be useful for screening. CT is helpful for clarifying the osseous situation and especially the fracture morphology. It is seldom necessary to carry out several examinations. If the case history is clear, it will suffice if the conventional radiograph correlates with the clinical findings; in cases of uncertainty (red flags), MRI examination will generally supply the necessary additional information for correct analysis and diagnosis. Comparison of the x-rays taken in standing and lying positions often reveals residual instabilities, which can be found in up to 40% of the patients [McKiernan 2003].

Indications and contraindications of vertebroplasty

The main indication for vertebroplasty is an osteoporotic fracture. The following conditions present clear indications:

- Osteoporotic fractures with corresponding pain lasting several weeks;
- Patients with very severe pain that keeps them in bed and which does not subside within 2–4 days after cement augmentation;
- Progressive collapse of one or several vertebrae accompanied by an increasing loss of posture; this should be treated with multi-level injections in one or several sessions;
- Pseudoarthroses with documented instability;
- In combination with an open stabilization for better anchorage of the implants and for protecting the adjacent vertebrae from fractures (see below).

Osteolyses in connection with tumors and metastases can be treated by means of cement augmentation. The complication risks and the results differ from the treatment of osteoporotic fractures.

Contraindications

- Pain not associated with a vertebral fracture;
- Infection;
- Coagulation disorder;
- Inadequate visualization on the image intensifier;
- Neurological deficit;
- An open intervention is indicated.

Surgical techniques and augmentation strategies

The presented technique is based on experience in over 500 patients with more than 2000 augmented vertebral bodies.

The operation is performed in three stages: 1. introduction of the filling cannula(e); 2. preparation of the cement; 3. cement application. The following instructions regarding the instruments should be observed: a) use of a guiding wire; b) use of large filling cannulae (8 gauge); c) use of special radiopaque cement with adequate viscosity; d) direct cement application by means of small disposable syringes.

Materials needed for performance of the operation

Local anesthesia (Mepivacaine 1%), 20 cc syringe with three-way tap for the cement distribution, 2 cc and 1 cc syringes for the cement injection. Guide wire 2 mm/20 cm 8 gauge disposable cannulae (Med Tech Gainsville Flordia). There are several high-radiopacity PMMA cements available for use in augmentation (Vertecem® Synthes, Vertebroplasty® DePuy Acromed, Osteopal®V Biomet-Merck, KyphX® Kyphon). There are various sets available on the market, such as the vertebroplasty set by Synthes® (Oberdorf, Switzerland).

The patient is positioned on a vacuum mattress, which allows optimal adjustment and offers the patient the greatest possible comfort. If the operation is performed under general anesthesia, we place the patient in hyperextension, so that in case of a possible instability a reduction can be achieved, or in order to support a restoration (lordoplasty) if this is intended (Fig. 89).

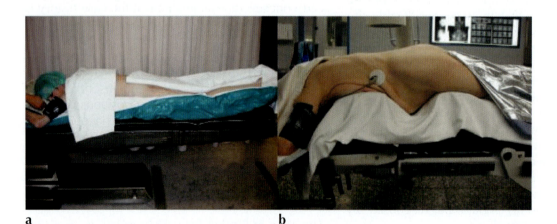

Fig. 89. a Positioning of patient for local anesthesia. A vacuum mattress is adjusted to ensure the comfort of the patient. **b** In general anesthesia the patient is positioned in a hyperextended position with a cushion to support the thorax and pelvis

Anesthesiological aspects

Percutaneous vertebroplasty, unlike lordo- and kyphoplasty, can usually be carried out under analgosedation. Local anesthesia of the puncture site and the periosteum does not suffice for the insertion of the guide wires and cannulae or for the cement injection. Maintenance of an adequate airway and sufficient spontaneous respiration during the analgosedation is crucial for patients lying in a prone position. Standard monitoring (ECG, indirect blood pressure reading and pulse oximetry) complemented by end-tidal CO_2 measurement via a nasal cannula is usually sufficient for most patients. Oxygen at 6–10 l/min is given via face mask. As vertebroplasty does not cause severe post-operative pain, an ultrashort-acting opiate is the preferred analgosedation. Infusion of remifentanil is started 10 minutes before the operation with a dosage of 0.05–0.1 µg/kg per min without administering a bolus. The infusion rate can then be increased until the respiratory frequency falls below 10 breaths/min or until the patient becomes somnolent, when the infusion rate must be reduced or the infusion temporarily stopped. Because of the very quick elimination of remifentanil, the respiratory depression quickly subsides again.

Bradycardia, hypotension and loss of consciousness could be indications of intravascular leakage of PMMA, therefore the blood pressure has to be monitored closely (every 2 min) during the injection of cement.

Lordoplasty and kyphoplasty, unlike pure vertebroplasty, are mostly performed under general anesthesia with endotracheal intubation.

Screening/imaging

An image intensifier with a large beam focus distance and very good image quality is needed for performance of the operation. Unhindered access in

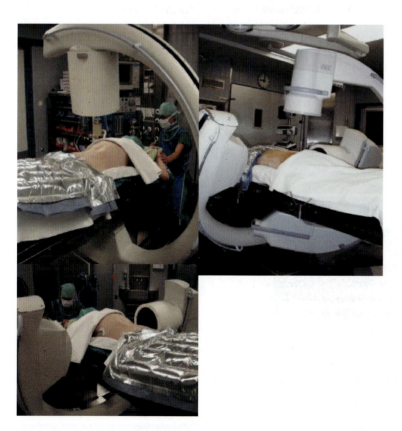

Fig. 90. Unhindered access of the image intensifier in the AP and lateral planes is essential. A C-arm with a long tube-camera distance is very helpful. The relevant vertebra has to be identified and marked before the operation field is sterilely draped. A biplanar exposure using two image intensifiers is possible, otherwise alternating AP and lateral views are necessary while injecting the cement

the PA and lateral planes is necessary. The section to be treated should be examined and marked before sterile draping the area. The operation should only be carried out if good visualization of the spine is possible; if otherwise, it should be refrained from, as is usually the case in fractures in the upper thoracic spine and may also be the case in the lower lumbar spine. A biplanar exposure using two image intensifiers can be an alternative (Fig. 90).

The vertebrae that are to be augmented are identified with the image intensifier. The x-ray has to be aligned exactly parallel with the endplates (in case of fractured vertebrae, the adjacent vertebrae are helpful as a reference). The vertebra is brought symmetrically into the AP projection. The access point for the cannula is defined on the skin on this basis and lies approx. 6 cm laterally of the midline (Fig. 91).

Placing the cannulae

A depot of local anesthesia is placed in the skin and periosteum at the entry point into the bone; 3–5 ml per puncture site. A guide wire is placed via a stab incision, converging caudally towards the spine. The wire is led by means of long forceps so that the operator's hands can be kept out of the x-ray path. In order to check the depth of the wire, a clamp is fixed approx. 3 cm above the skin level. At first bone contact, the position of the tip of the wire should be cranial and lateral of the pedicle projection. The guide wire is then driven further with hammer blows until the tip reaches the medial limitation of the pedicle (Fig. 91). If several vertebrae are being augmented, this step is repeated accordingly. The respective image with the position of the wire is saved in the image intensifier. The depth of the tip of the wire is now verified on the lateral view and should be at least at the height of the anterior wall of the vertebral body. The direction of the wire is corrected further if necessary and driven forward again by 1 cm. The filling cannulae are then pushed coaxially, by means of rotating movements, over the wire. The tip of the cannula should come to lie in the ventral half of the vertebral body. The guiding wire is removed, and the tip of the cannula is freed from bone with the blunt trocar (use hammer). This is also a helpful tactile check on the intraosseous situation (Fig. 92).

Preparation and injection of the cement

The cement is mixed as recommended by the manufacturer and filled into a 20 cc syringe; from there, it is filled into 2 cc and 1 cc syringes via a three-way tap. Alternatively an injection pistol can be used, though it is advisable to do without long connection tubes, since these offer high resistance and only allow the application of low-viscosity cement. The cement is not applied until the viscosity is high enough (Fig. 93), otherwise the flow cannot be controlled. In the drawn sample, the cement should be

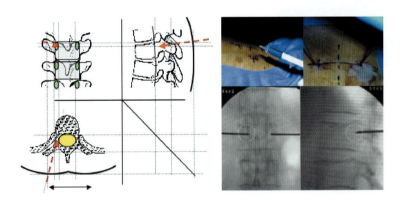

Fig. 91. Planning the placement of the guiding wire by means of an AP and a lateral projection: the surgeon must generate an axial projection from two lateral projections. The pedicles, endplates and vertebral body serve as landmarks. Depending on the pedicle size, the guiding wire is driven into the vertebral body either transpedicularly or converging parapedicularly. As soon as the tip of the wire has reached the medial limitation of the pedicle, it should at least touch the posterior wall of the vertebra on the lateral projection

Alternative methods to kyphoplasty: vertebroplasty – lordoplasty

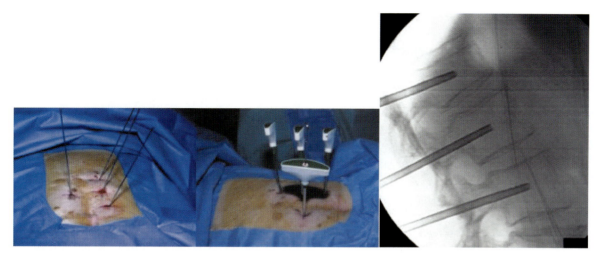

Fig. 92. After preliminary positioning of the guiding wires, the guiding cannulae are pushed over the wires under x-ray control and driven in at least as far as the ventral half of the vertebral body. The tips of the cannulae are freed from bone with the blunt trocar, which is also helpful as a tactile assessment of the intraosseous situation. In case of uncertainty regarding the position, a control x-ray in AP should be carried out

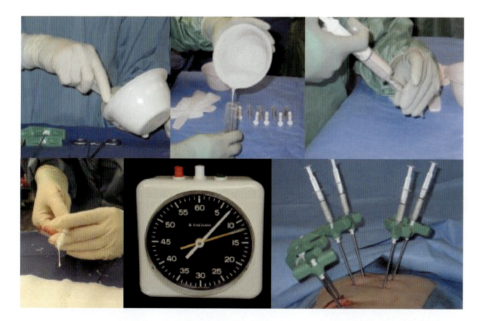

Fig. 93. Preparation of the cement (here Vertebroplastic®, DePuy): the components are mixed in a bowl with a spatula for 30 sec, and then after a further 30 sec, depending on the manufacturer, filled into a 20 cc syringe and left for another minute. After that the cement is filled into 2 cc syringes, which provide enough force to inject the cement (alternatively 1 cc syringes can be used). The cement has to have optimal viscosity before it is injected – which is when the cement no longer drips from the syringe. Thus Vertebroplastic® cement cannot be injected until 7 min after mixing

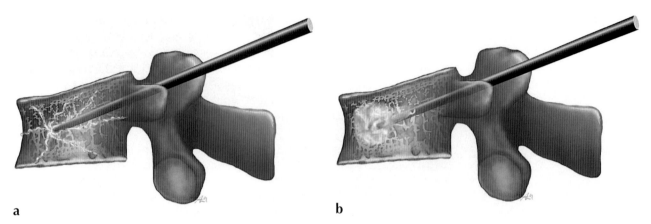

Fig. 94. Cement with low viscosity spreads uncontrolled within the spongiosa and shows a spidery picture (**a**), whereas highly viscous cement spreads more concentrically (**b**). As long as the viscosity of the cement is lower than the viscosity of the bone marrow, the cement cannot drive the bone marrow out

no longer dripping from the syringe but forming a thread. The viscosity of the cement is the decisive parameter in the risk of extravasation (Fig. 94a, b).

The cannula is carefully filled with cement and the flow can be observed within the cannula. The volume of the empty cannula should be known; for the cannula mentioned above it is 1.5 cc. As soon as the first cement becomes visible at the tip of cannula, the next cannula should be filled in the same manner. In bilateral access procedures the filling is carried out in stages so that both sides can be controlled. An intermittent image in the PA plane is recommended during the filling procedure. The filling itself is always carried out under lateral control with continuous image intensifier control (real time). If the filling goes correctly, the image of the cement should be that of a growing cloud (Fig. 95); if the cement advances to the periphery in a spidery manner at the beginning, the procedure must be temporarily interrupted. The cement hardens considerably faster in the body than at room temperature and after 45 sec it no longer spreads. The injection must be stopped in every case of cement extravasation. If, because of the increasing viscosity, it is no longer

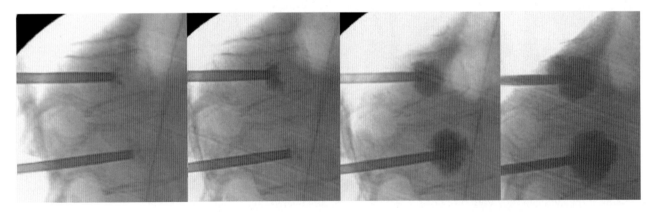

Fig. 95. The cement is injected under continuous control with an image intensifier. The condition of the cement at the tip of the cannula must be observed very closely: if the cement spreads away from the cannula in a particular direction, this means there is a connection to the venous system of the vertebral body. In this case another 45 sec should be waited before a little more cement is injected. In principle the cement should spread like a growing cloud and should be injected gradually. After 2 cc have been injected, an AP control should be carried out. If the injection resistance rises, the cement can be pressed from the cannula with the trocar. This technique permits controlled application of cement. The injection must be stopped if any signs of cement leakage show

possible to inject the cement via the syringe, the highly viscous cement can be pushed further with the trocar if need be, and possibly the cannula can be refilled again from the 1 cc syringes. The cements that are available have a long "working time" of approx. 5 minutes, making calm and controlled filling possible. The dorsal flow of cement (spinal canal) can be monitored very well; however, a second projection plane is needed for the flow in a lateral direction. It is necessary to wait until the cement has hardened before removing the filling cannulae. The cannula can then be loosened and removed with a slight turn; removal too early carries the risk of drawing cement filaments into the soft tissue. Hemorrhages at the puncture site are frequent and can cause temporary local irritation.

Strategies of the augmentation

In mild forms of osteoporosis, monosegmental injection of the fractured vertebra suffices. In acute fractures, bilateral access is recommended. If the filling on one side does not show the desired effect, it can usually be achieved on the other side (Fig. 96). In more severe cases of osteoporosis, augmentation of the adjacent cranial and caudal vertebrae is recommended, in addition to the fractured vertebra (Fig. 97). In this case the fracture is treated bilaterally and the connecting vertebrae monolaterally.

Both the natural course and the increased incidence of new fractures after augmentation justify this step [Lindsay 2001; Ross 1993; Uppin 2003; Kim 2004; Berlemann 2002]. Multi-level injection can be necessary in patients suffering from very severe osteoporosis and with a corresponding risk profile (steroid medication etc.). In general, this is carried out monolaterally, alternating between the left and right sides. A maximum of six vertebral bodies per session are augmented in 2 or 3 steps, injecting a maximum of 25–30 ml cement in order to avoid pulmonary strain as the result of washed out bone marrow (Fig. 98) [Heini 2005].

Correction of kyphosis: indication, technique, results

In the treatment of osteoporotic fractures it is necessary to re-establish the sagittal alignment if possible, as in classic treatment of fracture of the spine. However, because of the osteoporosis and the often poorer health of the patient, the technical possibilities are limited and may not allow this. Closed reduction should be tried in relevant cases of segmental kyphosis.

Vertebroplasty simply cements the status quo, and a correction is achieved only occasionally (Fig. 97). Apart from kyphoplasty, which may achieve correction to a certain extent, lordoplasty is

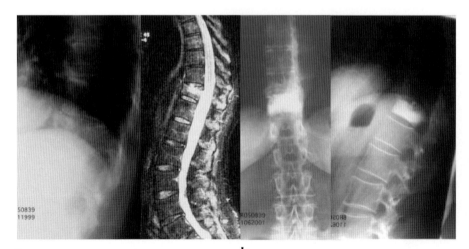

Fig. 96. A 70-year-old woman with compression fracture of T11 and in pain for 3 months. The MRI shows a persisting edema which indicates an acute fracture that has not yet healed (**a**). Immediate pain reduction after vertebroplasty, and further persisting pain reduction when presenting at follow-up (**b**). Follow-up after 1.5 years: the patient receives bisphosphonates as anti-osteoporotic therapy but does not take any analgesics

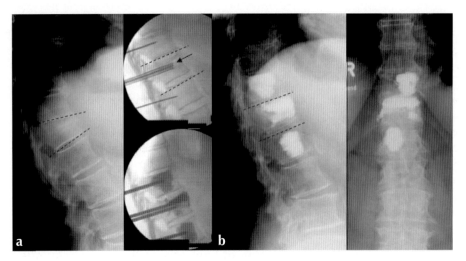

Fig. 97. Spontaneous reduction of a T12 fracture solely by positioning the patient. The x-ray taken in a standing positioning shows a relevant kyphosis (**a**). In the prone position, almost complete restoration of the vertebral body is seen, with a clearly visible defect zone (arrow). The filling pattern is characteristic for this defect (**b**). Almost completely preserved alignment of the spine when standing up. The adjoining vertebrae were augmented as a prophylactic measure

an alternative. In analogy with the principles of internal fixation, indirect repositioning is achieved with the support of the adjoining vertebrae via ligamentotaxis. Unlike kyphoplasty, where the initial reduction can frequently disappear after deflating the balloons, in lordoplasty the fractured vertebra can be augmented as a consequence of the existing prestressing.

Technique: The operation is carried out in three stages:

1. Bipedicular vertebroplasty of the adjoining cranial and caudal vertebral bodies (see above).
2. Reduction of the fractured vertebral body via the filling cannulae in place in the adjacent vertebrae.

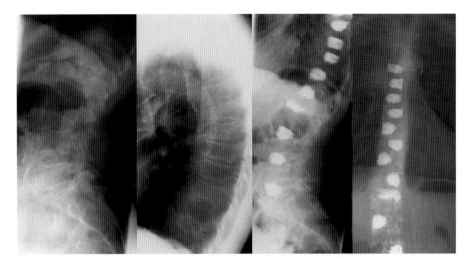

Fig. 98. A 68-year-old woman who received high-dosage steroid treatment for several years after heart transplantation. The patient complains of diffuse stress-related backache and episodes of rather severe pain. 7 cm height loss within the last 16 months. The x-ray shows multiple vertebral fractures within the region of the thoracic and lumbar spine. Vertebroplasty of T5 to L5 was carried out in three sessions of 45 minutes each. Further collapse was prevented; the patient subjectively felt an enormous improvement of the backache and a considerably more upright posture

3. Vertebroplasty of the reduced vertebral body. The patient is placed in a prone position, allowing the abdomen to hang freely, with a pad supporting the pelvis and sternum. The initial reduction achieved by mere positioning of the patient can be assessed in the lateral view on the image intensifier.

When inserting the Kirschner wire, the aim should be to achieve a slightly cranio-caudal direction in the cranial vertebral bodies, and a slightly caudo-cranial direction in the caudal ones (optimized reduction force). The depth of the six Kirschner wires is monitored in the lateral view. The cannulae are placed as described above, and both adjacent vertebral bodies are augmented. It is absolutely necessary that the trocars are introduced into the cannulae (to prevent bending) and are used to push another 1 ml of cement forward. Before the cement has hardened the cannulae are carefully advanced approx. 1 cm further, together with the trocars, so that they have a long fixation within the cement. After hardening of the cement (test the residual cement) a lordosing force is applied via the cannulae in place and, using the facet joints as a lever, the fractured vertebral body is restored in the sense of ligamentotaxis (anterior and posterior ligaments, anulus fibrosus). In principle, the reduction maneuver is the same as with an internal fixator [Dick 1987]. The reduction cannulae are either held with two Weber reduction pliers or fixed by means of a cross-bolt (blunt trocar) (Figs. 99–101). The vertebral body in the middle, being kept in a reduced state, is augmented with cement under continuous lateral image intensifier control. The fixation is not loosened until the cement has hardened. The cannulae can be removed easily with slight turns. In general the operation is carried out under general anesthesia in order to optimize the reduction (hyperlordosis, relaxation of the patient). If the bone quality is good, the adjoining cranial and caudal vertebral bodies do not have to be cemented. In selected cases this technique can be combined with kyphoplasty, which allows an even more efficient reduction.

Results: we have gathered experience with lordoplasty in over 70 patients, 31 of whom (7 m, 24 f) were recorded prospectively with a follow-up of at least a year. The average age of the fracture was 38 days. Persisting reduction of pain was achieved in 87% of the patients; the average improvement in all patients was 5 points (7.6 to 2.6) on a Visual Analog Scale from 0 to 10. Kyphosis correction of more than 10 degrees, assessed in the lateral radiograph in a standing position, was achieved in 57% of the patients. The average kyphosis correction in all patients was 12.4 degrees (Fig. 102). The material costs for the whole procedure amount to 400 euros. The

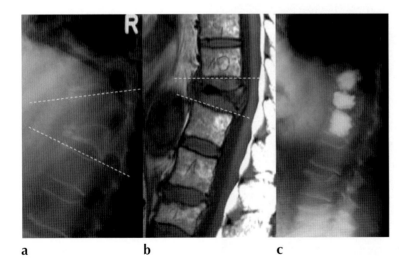

a b c

Fig. 99. A patient suffering from pain for 6 months after a T11 fracture (**a**). The pain occurs especially after standing up from lying. The MRI examination revealed collapse of T11 (**b**). Residual mobility could be detected, unlike on the x-ray taken in standing (**a**). Closed reduction (lordoplasty) was carried out. The post operative x-ray follow-up after 6 months shows a satisfactory situation with a good alignment (**c**) and a patient free from pain

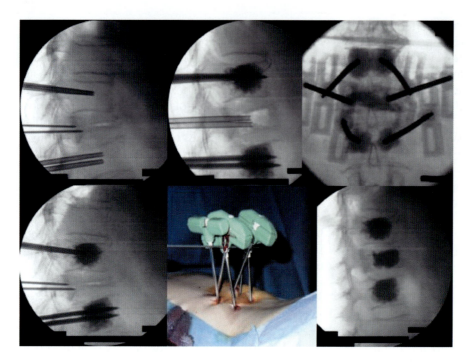

Fig. 100. The technique of lordoplasty corresponds to that of an indirect fracture reduction. The cranial and caudal cannulae are used as levers to raise the fractured vertebra. The defect after repositioning is clearly visible (*). The defect is cemented while maintaining the stress, and the cannulae are not removed until the cement has hardened

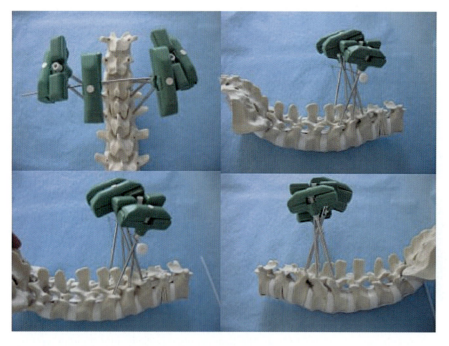

Fig. 101. Model of lordoplasty. The cannulae with lying trocar serve as levers to apply a lordosing moment. The cannulae are braced with a cross bolt

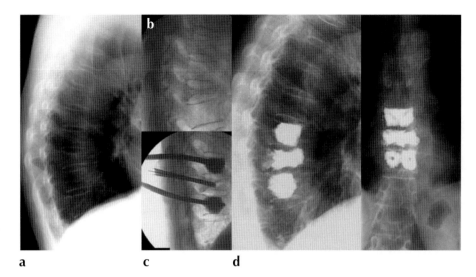

Fig. 102. A 76-year-old woman with fracture of T9 (**a**). The follow-up after 5 weeks shows almost complete collapse of the vertebral body (**b**). Relevant reduction of the vertebral body was achieved with lordoplasty (**c**). The follow-up in standing shows well maintained height of the vertebral body (**d**)

complications were partial root damage at L2 with a temporary sensorimotor deficit in one patient, and persisting instability in the movement segment after augmentation in two further patients, each resulting in open stabilization.

In summary, it can be stated that lordoplasty is an efficient, minimally invasive and economical method for restoring osteoporotic fractures, thus re-establishing the sagittal alignment of the spine at least partially. The indication for restoration is given for fractures with residual instability and relevant deformity. Fractures that are more than three months old can usually no longer be corrected, except in cases of pseudoarthrosis/osteonecrosis.

Combined surgical procedures

With the increasing incidence of osteoporotic fractures, the frequency of fractures with a complicated course involving spinal stenosis and/or severe malpositioning also increases [Kim 2003]. Open surgical procedure with stabilization of the affected movement segment is generally necessary in these cases [Natelson 1986]; however, anchorage of implants is often difficult. The combination of cement augmentation and pedicular stabilization provides an efficient option when technical difficulties seem otherwise unsolvable [Wuisman 2000; Moore 1997]. The pedicles are prepared in the normal manner, and then 7 gauge filling cannulae are introduced bilaterally and the cement applied to the vertebral body under image intensifier control. The pedicle screws are applied before the cement hardens, and the instrumentation can be completed as usual as soon as the cement has hardened. It is apparent that there is a great risk of fractures in the adjoining vertebrae in these patients, and it is inevitable that these are augmented percutaneously in the classic manner (Fig. 103). It is also possible to carry out percutaneous augmentation of the vertebral bodies beforehand. The preparation of the pedicle screws must then be carried out with a drill. PMMA can be easily treated. After drilling a hole with the 3.2 mm AO drill, 5 mm screws can be fixed without problems.

Limitations and complications

Even though cement augmentation is very successful, it should be borne in mind that the main problem of this technique is the extravasation of cement (embolization, spinal canal) [Bernhard 2003; Harrington 2001; Padovani 1999; Ratliff 2001; Ryu 2002; Scroop 2002; Tozzi 2002; Vasconcelos 2001; Yoo 2004]. The key to avoiding these potentially very dangerous and irreversible complications lies in the viscosity of the cement. Low-viscosity cement does not displace bone marrow and therefore flows primarily along vessel canals or fracture fissures. However, the flow cannot be controlled and thus

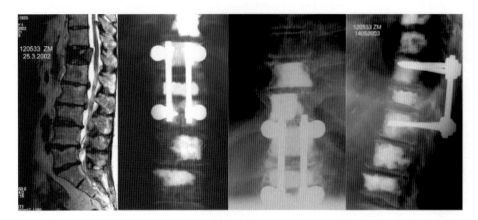

Fig. 103. A 69-year-old woman with unstable T12 fracture. The patient complained of numbness in both legs when standing up. Furthermore she was suffering from a basal plate impression fracture in the area of L3. The patient had steroid-induced osteoporosis and chronic obstructive lung disease, therefore a "small" operation with short stabilization and cementing of the adjacent vertebrae was carried out

the cement can be washed out by the blood flow within the vertebral body without hindrance. The higher the viscosity of the cement the safer is its application [Bohner 2003], though accordingly more strength is needed for the injection [Baroud 2004].

Safety can be optimized if the following parameters are observed: use of thick cannulae (smaller flow resistance), avoidance of long connection tubes (increased flow resistance, secondary flow of cement), direct cement injection with small syringes (good power transmission, controllable cement flow), waiting until the optimal viscosity has been reached.

Another aspect of which notice should be taken is the increased incidence of subsequent fractures after cement augmentation [Berlemann 2002; Grados 2000 Kim 2004; Uppin 2003]. Nevertheless, the natural course of the disease also shows an increased fracture risk that relates to the number of already fractured vertebrae [Lindsay 2001; Ross 1993] and this should be taken into account in the augmentation strategy (see above). The number of vertebrae treated per session should be restricted to six and the total volume of cement injected should not exceed 25–30 ml [Heini 2005; Heini and Orler 2004]. In the case of exacerbated pain, it is extremely important that the patient is evaluated again by the physicians dealing with the postoperative treatment.

Cement augmentation is not an efficient method for treating pronounced deformation; neither can percutaneous restoration methods (lordoplasty, kyphoplasty) help in fixed situations. A combined open intervention is indicated if the clinical situation requires this. Correct analysis of the fracture is essential; vertebroplasty alone cannot restore the stability of type B or C fractures.

References

Baroud G, Bohner M, Heini P, Steffen T (2004) Injection biomechanics of bone cements used in vertebroplasty. Biomed Mater Eng 14(4): 487–504

Barr JD, Barr MS, Lemley TJ, McCann RM (2000) Percutaneous vertebroplasty for pain relief and spinal stabilization. Spine 25(8): 923–8

Berlemann U, Ferguson SJ, Nolte LP, Heini PF (2002) Adjacent vertebral failure after vertebroplasty. A biomechanical investigation. J Bone Joint Surg Br 84(5): 748–52

Bernhard J, Heini PF, Villiger PM (2003) Asymptomatic diffuse pulmonary embolism caused by acrylic cement: an unusual complication of percutaneous vertebroplasty. Ann Rheum Dis 62(1): 85–6

Bohner M, Gasser B, Baroud G, Heini P (2003) Theoretical and experimental model to describe the injection of a polymethylmethacrylate cement into a porous structure. Biomaterials 24(16): 2721–30

Center JR, Nguyen TV, Schneider D, Sambrook PN, Eisman JA (1999) Mortality after all major types of osteoporotic fracture in men and women: an observational study. Lancet 353(9156): 878–82

Cortet B, Cotten A, Boutry N, Flipo RM, Duquesnoy B, Chastanet P, Delcambre B (1999) Percutaneous vertebroplasty in the treatment of osteoporotic vertebral compression fractures: an open prospective study. J Rheumatol 26(10): 2222–8

Cotten A, Dewatre F, Cortet B, Assaker R, Leblond D, Duquesnoy B, Chastanet P, Clarisse J (1996) Percutaneous vertebroplasty for osteolytic metastases and myeloma: effects of the percentage of lesion filling and the leakage of methyl methacrylate at clinical follow-up. Radiology 200(2): 525–30

Dick W (1987) The "fixateur interne" as a versatile implant for spine surgery. Spine 12(9): 882–900

Galibert P, Deramond H, Rosat P, Le Gars D (1987) Preliminary note on the treatment of vertebral angioma by percutaneous acrylic vertebroplasty. Neurochirurgie 33(2): 166–8

Grados F, Depriester C, Cayrolle G, Hardy N, Deramond H, Fardellone P (2000) Long-term observations of vertebral osteoporotic fractures treated by percutaneous vertebroplasty. Rheumatology (Oxford) 39(12): 1410–4

Harrington KD (2001) Major neurological complications following percutaneous vertebroplasty with polymethylmethacrylate: a case report. J Bone Joint Surg Am 83-A(7): 1070–3

Heini PF (2005) The current treatment-a survey of osteoporotic fracture treatment. Osteoporotic spine fractures: the spine surgeon's perspective. Osteoporos Int 16 [Suppl 2]: 85–92

Heini PF, Orler R (2004) Vertebroplasty in severe osteoporosis. Technique and experience with multi-segment injection. Orthopäde 33(1): 22–30

Heini PF, Walchli B, Berlemann U (2000) Percutaneous transpedicular vertebroplasty with PMMA: operative technique and early results. A prospective study for the treatment of osteoporotic compression fractures. Eur Spine J 9(5): 445–50

Jensen ME, Evans AJ, Mathis JM, Kallmes DF, Cloft HJ, Dion JE (1997) Percutaneous polymethylmethacrylate vertebroplasty in the treatment of osteoporotic vertebral body compression fractures: technical aspects. AJNR Am J Neuroradiol 18(10): 1897–904

Kim KT, Suk KS, Kim JM, Lee SH (2003) Delayed vertebral collapse with neurological deficits secondary to osteoporosis. Int Orthop 27(2): 65–9

Kim SH, Kang HS, Choi JA, Ahn JM (2004) Risk factors of new compression fractures in adjacent vertebrae after percutaneous vertebroplasty. Acta Radiol 45(4): 440–5

Legroux-Gerot I, Lormeau C, Boutry N, Cotten A, Duquesnoy B, Cortet B (2004) Long-term follow-up of vertebral osteoporotic fractures treated by percutaneous vertebroplasty. Clin Rheumatol 23(4): 310–7

Lindsay R (2001) Risk of new vertebral fracture in the year following a fracture. Jama 285(1): 320–323

McKiernan F, Jensen R, Faciszewski T (2003) The dynamic mobility of vertebral compression fractures. J Bone Miner Res 18(1): 24–9

Melton LJ, 3rd, Kan SH, Frye MA, Wahner HW, O'Fallon WM, Riggs BL (1989) Epidemiology of vertebral fractures in women. Am J Epidemiol 129(5): 1000–11

Moore DC, Maitra RS, Farjo LA, Graziano GP, Goldstein SA (1997) Restoration of pedicle screw fixation with an in situ setting calcium phosphate cement. Spine 22(15): 1696–705

Natelson SE (1986) The injudicious laminectomy. Spine 11(9): 966–9

Padovani B, Kasriel O, Brunner P, Peretti-Viton P (1999) Pulmonary embolism caused by acrylic cement: a rare complication of percutaneous vertebroplasty. AJNR Am J Neuroradiol 20(3): 375–7

Peh WC, Gilula LA, Peck DD (2002) Percutaneous vertebroplasty for severe osteoporotic vertebral body compression fractures. Radiology 223(1): 121–6

Ratliff J, Nguyen T, Heiss J (2001) Root and spinal cord compression from methylmethacrylate vertebroplasty. Spine 26(13): E300–2

Ross PD, Genant HK, Davis JW, Miller PD, Wasnich RD (1993) Predicting vertebral fracture incidence from prevalent fractures and bone density among non-black, osteoporotic women. Osteoporos Int 3(3): 120–6

Ryu KS, Park CK, Kim MC, Kang JK (2002) Dose-dependent epidural leakage of polymethylmethacrylate after percutaneous vertebroplasty in patients with osteoporotic vertebral compression fractures. J Neurosurg 96 [1 Suppl]: 56–61

Scroop R, Eskridge J, Britz GW (2002) Paradoxical cerebral arterial embolization of cement during intraoperative vertebroplasty: case report. AJNR Am J Neuroradiol 23(5): 868–70

Tozzi P, Abdelmoumene Y, Corno AF, Gersbach PA, Hoogewoud HM, von Segesser LK (2002) Management of pulmonary embolism during acrylic vertebroplasty. Ann Thorac Surg 74(5): 1706–8

Uppin AA, Hirsch JA, Centenera LV, Pfiefer BA, Pazianos AG, Choi IS (2003) Occurrence of new vertebral body fracture after percutaneous vertebroplasty in patients with osteoporosis. Radiology 226(1): 119–24

Vasconcelos C, Gailloud P, Martin JB, Murphy KJ (2001) Transient arterial hypotension induced by polymethylmethacrylate injection during percutaneous vertebroplasty. J Vasc Interv Radiol 12(8): 1001–2

Weill A, Chiras J, Simon JM, Rose M, Sola-Martinez T, Enkaoua E (1996) Spinal metastases: indications for and results of percutaneous injection of acrylic surgical cement. Radiology 199(1): 241–7

Wuisman PI, Van Dijk M, Staal H, Van Royen BJ (2000) Augmentation of (pedicle) screws with calcium apatite cement in patients with severe progressive osteoporotic spinal deformities: an innovative technique. Eur Spine J 9(6): 528–33

Yoo KY, Jeong SW, Yoon W, Lee J (2004) Acute respiratory distress syndrome associated with pulmonary cement embolism following percutaneous vertebroplasty with polymethylmethacrylate. Spine 29(14): E294–7

Zoarski GH, Snow P, Olan WJ, Stallmeyer MJ, Dick BW, Hebel JR, De Deyne M (2002) Percutaneous vertebroplasty for osteoporotic compression fractures: quantitative prospective evaluation of long-term outcomes. J Vasc Interv Radiol 13(2 Pt 1): 139–48

Chapter 12

Injectable cements for vertebroplasty and kyphoplasty

M. Bohner

In all bone augmentation procedures such as vertebroplasty and kyphoplasty, the cement plays a key role. However, until a few years ago very little had been done to optimize the properties of the cement; in fact, very little had been done to understand which properties the cement should have. The aim of the present manuscript is first to give a general introduction to cements, mostly PMMA and CPC, and second to review the most recent findings in the field.

Various cements

In the present section, the general properties of PMMA and CPC cements are described, the two cements are critically compared, and new cements and cement developments are briefly reviewed.

PMMA cements: the first cement that was used for a bone augmentation procedure was a poly(methyl methacrylate) (PMMA) cement [Galibert et al. 1987]. This cement consists of several ingredients that all have their importance [Kühn 2000]:

(i) methyl methacrylate (MMA) monomer (transparent liquid; MW = 100 g/mole) that will eventually react to form PMMA. The heat released by the latter reaction is very great, i.e. close to 57 kJ/mole, whereas the specific heat of PMMA is relatively low, i.e. close to 1.46 J/(g·K) [Vallo 2002]. As a result, the heat released during the reaction is large enough to potentially heat up the cement by several hundred degrees during setting.

(ii) a PMMA powder (or copolymer) that is used as a filler material, hence decreasing the total heat released per cement volume as well as reducing the shrinkage during setting (−21% for pure MMA).

(iii) a radio-opacifier to make sure that the cement can be seen radiographically (radio-opacifier in-

cluded in or added to the PMMA powder). Typical powders are $BaSO_4$ and ZrO_2.

(iv) some additives to initiate the polymerization reaction, usually dibenzoyl peroxide (generally included in or added to the PMMA powder) and N,N-dimethyl-p-toluidine (generally included in the liquid phase)

(v) other additives such as stabilizers, inhibitors, radical catchers, coloring agents and antibiotics.

In commercial formulations, the ratio between powder and liquid component is typically close to 2:3. In addition, the radio-opacifier content can easily reach 30%. For example, Osteopal V (Biomet) contains in the powder component 14.16 g PMMA (40.0w% of the total cement weight), 11.70 g ZrO_2 (33.1w%), 0.14 g benzoyl peroxide (0.4w%) and chlorophyll (coloring agent); in the liquid component 9.2 g MMA (26w%), 0.19 g N,N-dimethyl-p-toluidine (0.5%) and chlorophyll. As the MMA content is relatively small, shrinkage and heat release of commercial cement formulations are much lower than those of pure MMA cement.

Importantly, the curing (setting or hardening) reaction of PMMA cements is a polymerization reaction, i.e. small monomers react together to form increasingly long polymer chains. Hardening occurs via the entanglement of the polymer chains, and the reaction stops when no more MMA monomers are present. The final porosity of the cement is close to zero.

In the early days, PMMA cements used for vertebroplasty were modified to better fulfill the requirements of the application. In particular, the powder-to-liquid ratio was reduced to prolong the injection period, and more radio-opacifier was added to increase the radiological contrast. These changes considerably modified cement properties such as viscosity, setting time, monomer release and mechanical properties. As there was no cement accepted for vertebral bone augmentation procedures, these changes were made but the cements were used at the patients' and clinicians' own risk (off-label use). Nowadays there are cements designed specifically for the application (e.g. Kyph'X, Osteofirm, Osteopal V, Spineplex, Synicem VTP, Vertebroplastic, Vertecem) and therefore their use is recommended.

Calcium phosphate cements (CPCs): these were discovered two decades ago by LeGeros [LeGeros et al. 1982] and Brown and Chow [Brown and Chow 1983]. Since then, these cements have proved to be attractive bone substitute materials [Constantz et al. 1995]. The first *in vitro* attempt to use CPC for the augmentation of osteoporotic bone was made more than a decade ago [Bohner et al. 1992], and a few years later the first *in vitro* use for intravertebral reconstruction was proposed [Schildhauer et al. 1995].

CPCs generally consist of an aqueous solution and a powder that typically contains several calcium phosphate compounds. Upon mixing, the powder dissolves in the aqueous solution and new crystals form (precipitate), the reaction proceeding until all reactive calcium phosphate compounds have reacted. Cement hardening occurs with the entanglement of calcium phosphate crystals (Fig. 104), hence leading to a highly porous structure. The final product has a porosity close to 40–60%, with pores ranging typically from 0.1 to 10 μm. It is noteworthy that CPCs are mechanically much stronger in compression than in tension or shear, because entangled crystals are not well bonded. Compressive strength is typically 5 to 10 times larger than the tensile strength.

There are two types of CPC: apatite (e.g. hydroxyapatite, $Ca_5(PO_4)_3(OH)$) and brushite (dicalcium phosphate dihydrate; $CaHPO_4 \cdot 2H_2O$), depending on the end-product of the setting reaction [Bohner 2000]. Most of the CPCs sold on the market belong to the first category e.g. α-BSM, Biopex, BoneSource, Calcibon, Cementek, Embarc, Kyphos, Mimix, Norian, Rebone. In recent months, a few brushite CPCs have been tested clinically: chronOS Inject, Eurobone and VitalOS. The main difference between apatite and brushite CPCs lies in their solubility and hence resorption rate: brushite is much more soluble than apatite, so brushite CPCs in principle resorb faster than apatite CPCs.

Differences between PMMA and CPC: as CPCs are the main candidates to replace PMMA in vertebroplasty, it is of interest to describe the main differences between CPC and PMMA cements. Some of the differences are very important (Table 9) and four of these are described here. Firstly, PMMA cements are hydrophobic, whereas CPC are hydrophilic. Thus the setting reaction of PMMA is hardly affected by body fluids, in contrast to that of CPC where cement disintegration might occur, leading to the release of a very large number of micro- and nanoparticles in the close environment of the cement and into blood. Secondly, the setting reaction occurs much faster in PMMA cements than in CPCs. As a result, reaction heat is released much faster from PMMA cements than from CPCs, leading to a much larger temperature increase in the former. So, even though CPCs are sometimes as exothermic as PMMA, CPC can be considered to set isothermally. Thirdly, CPCs are very fragile materials. In particular, the shear and tensile properties of CPCs are much lower than those of PMMA cements. However, in principle, these low properties should not affect the outcome of vertebral bone augmentation procedures, because it is generally accepted that the most important mechanical property to consider in vertebral bone augmentation is the compressive strength. Moreover, it is known that the compressive strength of CPC is much greater than that of cancellous bone. Nevertheless, clinicians have related negative results of vertebral bone augmentation performed with CPC to the low shear properties (cement cracking). Clearly, it is necessary to collect more data on the use of CPC in vertebral bone augmentation. Fourth-

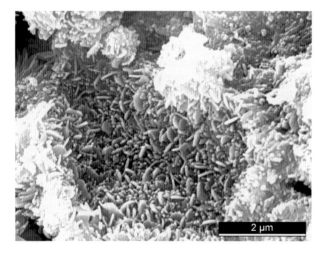

Fig. 104. Typical structure of an apatite CPC showing the entanglement of small apatite crystals

Table 9. Summary of the main features of PMMA and calcium phosphate cements

	PMMA cement	CPC
Hydrophilicity	Hydrophobic	Hydrophilic
Injectability	Excellent	Critical
Setting time	< 20 minutes	< 20 minutes
Setting rate	Very fast	Slow
Temperature change	Large	Negligible
Tensile strength	> 50 MPa [2]	< 15 MPa
Compressive strength	> 70 MPa [2]	< 100 MPa
Porosity	Close to 0%	40–60%
Pore diameter	–	0.1–10 µm
Resorption	No	Little to great
Bone-cement contact	Limited	Excellent

ly, in contrast to PMMA cements, CPCs are resorbable and therefore should be replaced by bone and not simply be resorbed. At present, it is not clear how fast CPCs resorb and how much bone forms after CPC resorption in patients with osteoporosis.

Other cements: there are few new approaches in the field of polymeric and ceramic cements. One recent development in the field of methacrylate cements is represented by Cortoss, which has a more complex composition than traditional PMMA cements. The presence of three specific methacrylate components is intended to reduce release of toxic monomer and improve the mechanical properties in comparison with PMMA cements. In addition, a high ceramic fraction provides good radiological contrast and helps to reduce the extent of the temperature increase during setting. However, this cement is stiffer than PMMA cements and also tends to be very liquid compared with the requirements set by vertebroplasty (Viscosity > 100 Pa·s). Another recent development is a non-resorbable cement based on a mixture of functional thiols, acrylic molecules, a reaction starter, a thixotropic agent and barium sulfate (32w%) [Zamparo 2004]. This cement has a compressive strength close to 30–40 MPa (cancellous bone has a value lower than 10 MPa) and an E-modulus lower than that of cancellous bone (close to 70 MPa, compared with 100–

500 MPa for cancellous bone and more than 1 GPa for PMMA cement). As a result, augmentation of a vertebral body with this cement does not significantly affect bone compliance, which might reduce the risk of adjacent vertebral fractures. In the field of ceramic cements, the most advanced project appears to be a non-resorbable cement based on calcium aluminate that has very low porosity and hence very large mechanical properties [Axen et al. 2004]. Indeed flexural and compressive strengths close to 30–50 MPa and 150–180 MPa, respectively, have been reported. The E-modulus is unfortunately very high, close to 10–12 GPa (cancellous bone: 0.1–0.5 GPa).

Cement properties for vertebroplasty

In the last few years, general understanding about the necessary and adequate properties of cements for vertebral bone augmentation procedures has been widely improved. Parameters of importance are the cement handling, viscosity, injection time, injectability, radio-opacity, setting time, exothermic heat, mechanical properties, blood clotting properties and monomer release. This section reviews these parameters.

Handling: procedures such as cement mixing and syringe filling should be easy and reliable. In that respect, most cements fulfill these requirements, even though improvements could be made.

Viscosity: cement viscosity is a very important parameter for the application. The viscosity defines the injection pressure but more importantly the risk of extravasation [Bohner et al. 2003; Breusch et al. 2002], which decreases with an increase of the cement viscosity. It is therefore important to find an adequate balance between a high cement viscosity that reduces extravasation risks and a low viscosity that enables low injection forces. The use of an adequate injection system is then required. Cement viscosity in the range of 100–1000 Pa·s appears to be ideal.

Injection time: Ideally, a cement should have a constant viscosity in the range previously mentioned. Unfortunately, cement viscosity is not a constant value: after a decrease in the first seconds after mixing, the viscosity increases considerably during curing, eventually leading to hardening. The viscosity should be high enough to prevent extravasation, therefore it is important to define an adequate injection window. At present, none of the cement manufacturers provides information on adequate cement viscosity, so many clinicians inject the cement too early in a too liquid state. In addition, none of the manufacturers provides a way of determining adequate viscosity in the OR, even though cement viscosity depends very strongly on temperature. Clearly, there is at the moment a strong need to improve the information given to clinicians.

Injectability: here, the injectability of a cement is defined as the ability of the cement to be injected without phase separation between fluid and powder. PMMA cements are easily injectable, in contrast to CPCs which tend to phase-separate or filter-press: above a certain injection pressure, the liquid phase is injected faster than the powder phase, eventually leading to plugging. When plugging occurs (e.g. in bone), injection of the cement is no longer possible. Several approaches can be used to improve CPC injectability; for example, an increase of the liquid-to-powder ratio [Bohner and Baroud 2005]. However, the best approach appears to be the addition of a small amount of polymer gel (e.g. 0.5–1.0% sodium hyaluronate gel) into the mixing liquid, so that interparticle contacts are lubricated without decreasing the cement viscosity.

Radio-opacity: Unlike CPCs, PMMA cements have hardly any radiological contrast; however, both types of cement require additional contrast. For PMMA cements, the choice is relatively easy because these cements are not resorbable, thus all radio-opaque non- or poorly-soluble powders such as metal salts ($BaSO_4$, ZrO_2, $SrCO_3$) or metal powders (Ti, Ta, W) may be used. For CPCs, the problem is more difficult. CPCs are indeed slowly resorbable, therefore all added powders are released over time. Most metallic salts are barely soluble ($SrCO_3$) or fully insoluble ($BaSO_4$, ZrO_2), which means that billions of small radio-opaque particles will be released over time; this might represent a biocompatibility hazard and needs to be looked at carefully. Another possibility is to increase the solid content of the cement by increasing the powder-to-liquid ratio; this can be done but has limited efficacy and reduces cement injectability. It is also possible to add a liquid radiological contrast agent such as iodine-based aqueous solutions, but unfortunately a small fraction of the population is allergic to iodide (death casualties have been reported).

Setting time: the setting time of a cement is defined as the time required for the cement to reach a given mechanical strength. This property can be modified quite easily, so that most cements designed for vertebral bone augmentation have a setting time in the range of 5–20 minutes. It is noteworthy that the setting rate of the cement is more difficult to control: as soon as the setting reaction starts, the reaction cannot be slowed down or accelerated. Typically, PMMA cements harden very fast (20–30 minutes), whereas CPCs harden rather slowly (100% of the mechanical strength after 5–10 hours).

Exothermic heat: the reason for relief of pain following vertebral bone augmentation procedure has been topic of controversy. Two main explanations have been proposed. Firstly, pain relief results from the mechanical stabilization of the vertebral body; this is the most frequently mentioned explanation nowadays. Secondly, pain relief results from the necrosis of nerves as a result of the large amount of heat released from the cement; in that respect, it would be important to always use very exothermic and fast-setting cements, such as PMMA cements.

Several studies have been published on the thermic effect of PMMA cements after vertebral bone augmentation (e.g. [Belkoff and Molloy 2003]). To better understand these studies, it is important to note that heat/exothermic release and temperature increase during setting are related phenomena but are not the same thing: the temperature increase depends not only on the rate of heat release but also on the rate of heat dispersion. In other words, very exothermic cement reactions do not necessarily lead to a temperature increase if the rate of heat release is very low (for example in CPCs) or if heat dispersion is very good. Heat dispersion is favored (i) when the cement is in contact with a material with a high heat conductance (such as a metallic implant), (ii) when the cement is in contact with a flowing liquid (e.g. blood), and (iii) when the cement piece has a high specific surface (ratio between cement surface and cement volume).

Mechanical properties: the mechanical effect of vertebral bone augmentation has been investigated intensively. A particular point of interest is the potential negative effect of bone augmentation on fractures of adjacent vertebrae [Berlemann et al. 2002]. Even though finite element models suggest that vertebrae adjacent to a vertebra augmented with a stiff material such as PMMA or CPC are submitted to higher loads than normal [Polikeit et al. 2003; Baroud et al. 2003], it is not clear how important this effect is. Assuming that cement stiffness is a very important parameter and should be reduced, a problem occurs because it is difficult to reduce the stiffness of PMMA cements or CPCs. The only possibility is to decrease the cement porosity, and

Injectable cements for vertebroplasty and kyphoplasty

this approach has been proposed by Bisig et al. [Bisig et al. 2003], who incorporated an aqueous phase into a PMMA cement paste based on the idea of DeWijn [De Wijn 1976]. Stiffness in the range of that of cancellous bone could be obtained with 40% aqueous fraction. However, this approach does not work with CPCs, because these cements are already highly porous. An alternative could be to use new types of material, such as the compliant cement mentioned here. A second point of interest concerning the mechanical properties of cements are the fatigue properties, particularly those of CPCs, since these are fragile materials and have much lower mechanical properties than PMMA cements. To date, there is to our knowledge only one study on the fatigue properties of CPC [Gisep et al. 2004]. Again, more work needs to be done, perhaps also in combination with *in vivo* studies.

Blood clotting: this topic has received considerable attention in the last 12 months following the abstract of Bernards et al. [Bernards et al. 2004], who demonstrated that injection of CPC into the blood stream of pigs provoked rapid embolization and death. Related results were obtained in an *in vitro* study by Axen et al. [Axen et al. 2004]. The latter authors observed that CPC and calcium sulfate led to blood clotting, whereas a calcium aluminate cement [Axen et al. 2004] and PMMA did not provoke any clotting. Another study devoted to PMMA confirmed the absence or limited effect of PMMA cements on blood clotting [Blinc et al. 2004]. There are several possible explanations for the negative effect of CPC on clotting; for example, the release of Ca ions – these play a very important role in the clotting cascade. However, the most likely explanation appears to be that release of calcium phosphate particles from the cement into the blood stream triggers blood clotting. The fact that PMMA cements are hydrophobic (water repellent) whereas CPC are hydrophilic could explain the difference between these materials. Additional information is required to confirm the present interpretation of the data.

Monomer release: the release of MMA from PMMA cements during setting has been related to severe hypotension caused by action on vascular smooth muscle [Kim and Ritter 1972; Karlsson et al. 1995]. At present there is a large amount of data available in the field of hip arthroplasty but little in the field of vertebral bone augmentation. Despite the fact that the injected volume of cements is lower in vertebral bone augmentation than in hip ar-

throplasty, for several reasons it is of great importance to determine how much monomer is released from PMMA cements during setting. Four main reasons can be mentioned: (i) the liquid-to-powder ratios of cements used for vertebroplasty are generally lower than those used in hip arthroplasty, which should lead to more monomer release; (ii) the setting times of cements used for vertebroplasty are generally longer than those used in hip arthroplasty, which should lead to more monomer release; (iii) vertebral bodies are very well irrigated bones, and (iv) vertebral bodies are in very close proximity to the heart.

Conclusions

In the first part of this chapter, the general properties of PMMA cements and CPCs were presented and discussed; new cements and cement developments were briefly mentioned. In the second part, the various cement properties that have to be adapted for vertebral bone augmentation were discussed, and properties such as cement handling, viscosity, injection time, injectability, radio-opacity, setting time, exothermic heat, mechanical properties, blood clotting properties and monomer release were considered. The main conclusions are that there is probably room for new cements with better adapted properties, such as high compliance, and that despite recent work much needs to be done to define adequate properties of cements used in vertebral bone augmentation.

References

Axen N, Ahnfelt N-O, Persson T, Hermansson L, Sanchez J, Larsson R (2004) Clotting behavior of orthopaedic cements in human blood. Proceedings of the 9th annual meeting "Ceramics, cells and tissues", Faenza

Axen N, Persson T, Bjorklund K, Engqvist H, Hermansson L (2004) An injectable bone void filler cement based on Ca-aluminate. Key Eng Mater 254–256: 265–8

Baroud G, Nemes J, Heini P, Steffen T (2003) Load shift of the intervertebral disc after a vertebroplasty: a finite-element study. Eur Spine J 12(4): 421–6

Belkoff SM, Molloy S (2003) Temperature measurement during polymerization of polymethylmethacrylate cement used for vertebroplasty. Spine 28(14): 1555–9

Berlemann U, Ferguson SJ, Nolte LP, Heini PF (2002) Adjacent vertebral failure after vertebroplasty – A biomechanical investigation. J Bone Joint Surg-Br 84B(5): 748–52

Bernards CM, Chapman JR, Mirza SK. Lethality of embolized norian bone cement varies with the time between mixing and embolization. Proceedings of the 50th Annual Meeting of the Orthopaedic Research Society(ORS), San Fransisco, p 254

Bisig A, Bohner M, Schneider E (2003) Biomechanical adaptation of PMMA vertebroplasty in osteoporotic spines. Proceedings of the GRIBOI meeting 2003, Baltimore, USA (Talk)

Blinc A, Bozic M, Vengust R, Stegnar M (2004) Methylmethacrylate bone cement surface does not promote platelet aggregation or plasma coagulation in vitro. Thromb Res 114(3): 179–84

Bohner M, Baroud G (2005) Injectability of calcium phosphate pastes. Biomaterials 26(13): 1553–63

Bohner M, Gasser B, Baroud G, Heini P (2003) Theoretical and experimental model to describe the injection of a polymethylmethacrylate cement into a porous structure. Biomaterials 24(6): 2721–30

Bohner M, Lemaître J, Cordey J, Gogolewski S, Ring TA, Perren SM (1992) Potential use of biodegradable bone cement in bone surgery: holding strength of screws in reinforced osteoporotic bone. Orthopaedic Trans 16: 401–2

Bohner M (2000) Calcium orthophosphates in medicine: from ceramics to calcium phosphate cements. Injury 31S(4): 37–47

Breusch S, Heisel C, Mueller J, Borchers T, Mau H (2002) Influence of cement viscosity on cement interdigitation and venous fat content under in vivo conditions. Acta Orthop Scand 73(4): 409–15

Brown WE, Chow LC (1983) A new calcium phosphate setting cement. J Dental Res 62: 672

Constantz BR, Ison IC, Fulmer MT, Poser RD, Smith ST, VanWagoner M, Ross J, Goldstein SA, Jupiter JB, Rosenthal DI (1995) Skeletal repair by in situ formation of the mineral phase of bone. Science 267: 1796–9

De Wijn JR (1976) Poly(methyl methacrylate) – aqueous phase blends: in situ curing porous materials. J Biomed Mater Res 10: 625–35

Galibert P, Deramond H, Rosat P, Le Gars D (1987) Preliminary note on the treatment of vertebral angioma by percutaneous acrylic vertebroplasty. Neurochir 33(2): 166–8

Gisep A, Kugler S, Wahl D, Rahn B (2004) Mechanical characterisation of a bone defect model filled with ceramic cements. J Mater Sci Mater Med 15(10): 1065–71

Karlsson J, Wendling W, Chen D, Zelinsky J, Jeevanandam V, Hellman S, Carlsson C (1995) Methylmethacrylate monomer produces direct relaxation of vascular smooth muscle in vitro. Acta Anaesthesiol Scand 39(5): 685–9

Kim KC, Ritter MA (1972) Hypotension associated with methyl methacrylate in total hip arthroplasties. Clin Orthop 88: 154–60

Kühn KD (2000) Bone cements: Up-to-date comparison of physical and chemical properties of commercial materials. Springer, Berlin Heidelberg

LeGeros RZ, Chohayeb A, Shulman A (1982) Apatitic calcium phosphates: possible dental restorative materials. J Dental Res 61: 343

Polikeit A, Nolte LP, Ferguson SJ (2003) The effect of cement augmentation on the load transfer in an osteoporotic functional spinal unit: Finite-element analysis. Spine 28(10): 991–6

Schildhauer TA, Bennett AP, Tomin E, Wright TM, Lane JM, Poser RD, Constantz BR (1995) Biomechanical evaluation of a new method for intra-vertebral body reconstruction with an injectable in situ setting carbonated apatite. Combined Orthopaedic Res Soc Meeting, San Diego, California, p 237

Vallo CI (2002) Theoretical prediction and experimental determination of the effect of mold characteristics on temperature and monomer conversion fraction profiles during polymerization of a PMMA-based bone cement. J Biomed Mater Res 63(5): 627–42

Zamparo E (2004) Novel biocompliant material for vertebroplasty. Vertebroplasty Course, Geneva, Switzerland

Chapter 13

Physiotherapeutic treatment after balloon kyphoplasty – aspects and concepts

Silke Becker

A new surgical treatment requires correspondingly adapted postoperative physiotherapy treatment, opening new approaches based on the latest scientific findings.

Osteoporosis is a disease for which diagnosis and therapy have the highest priority, requiring cooperation of all disciplines involved, especially if an osteoporotic vertebral body fracture (VBF) has already occurred.

Though surgery can achieve a proper reconstruction of a fracture, it cannot influence osteoporosis in the sense of healing, but is merely one element within an interdisciplinary treatment regimen.

Reduced bone mass and osteoporotic fractures cannot be treated by drugs alone, and merely treating patients with vertebroplasty or balloon kyphoplasty without offering or developing an appropriate concept for postoperative treatment is also questionable. Physiotherapy plays an important role in treatment after VBFs and in prevention of further fractures. The positive effect of physiotherapy in patients suffering from osteoporosis without VBF has been scientifically well documented [Bérard 1997; Wolff 1999; Sinaki 2002], and although there is no evaluated treatment concept for osteoporotic patients after minimally invasive surgery of a VBF, this group of patients should not be deprived of adequate therapy.

Every posture and movement of the body involves aspects of balance. Posture and equilibrium change negatively with advancing age and correlate with the risk of falling [Lynn 1997]. Patients with distinct kyphosis are especially at risk; in general it can be said that the more pronounced the kyphosis, the worse the balance and the greater the risk of falling. Osteoporotic patients suffering from a VBF are thus particularly endangered. Furthermore, movement behavior is changed in the sense of atax-

ia, which causes nonphysiological falling behavior, with increased risk of fracture as a result of the decreased bone density. In connection with this, Bös and Brehm [1998] draw attention to physical equilibrium being an important prerequisite for the execution and mastering of physical activities in everyday life. A balance disorder leads to an increased incidence of falling and to fear of further accidents, resulting in avoidance behavior in relevant situations or to inactivity [Skelton 2001]. In this sense, training the balance is of special significance since the sense of equilibrium is regarded as the quintessential coordinative active competence, which in turn plays a large part in increase of everyday competence (quality of life).

Thus the avoidance of kyphosis can be seen as active prophylaxis against falling.

The increased risk of falling is not the only important reason to avoid kyphosis; the mobility of other joints is also influenced negatively by kyphosis. The shoulder joints in particular are considerably reduced in their function, with the consequence that patients can no longer pull their clothes over their head on their own, and may also have great difficulties with their personal hygiene. The mobility of the cervical spine is also considerably limited, leading to a restricted field of vision, which results in increasing uncertainty and increased risk of falling.

Furthermore, as a consequence of the ribs drawing near to the iliac crest, the abdominal cavity is reduced, i.e. the internal organs are being compressed. This can lead to a change in organ function, e.g. in the colon, leading to constipation, and also leads to an increase of pressure on the pelvic floor. Since the pelvic floor is frequently the weakest link in the chain, it can thus lead to incontinence, especially in women (see below).

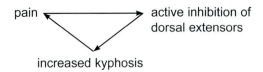

Fig. 105. Vicious circle of pain – muscles – posture

Only one study has examined and supported the relation between spinal deformity and prolapsed organs of the pelvis [Mattox 2000].

Kyphosis not only presents a static problem but can also be partly responsible for pain. The patient does not notice the change in static at first, as the course is progressive and he/she has time to adapt to the new situation. The pain, however, directly influences the dorsal muscles and thus encourages a worsening of the kyphotic malposition (Fig. 105).

Patients cannot actively interrupt this viscous circle of pain – muscles – posture on their own and so the individual factors increase mutually. Merely activating the dorsal muscles cannot stop the progress of an already existing pathological kyphosis. Quite often the only thing that helps is for the patient to wear a corset which, however, also has many disadvantages. In addition to the low compliance with patients, a corset supports muscle deactivation and can therefore be counterproductive with respect to the kyphosis. If possible, it is important to avoid the wearing of a rigid corset over a long time period [Sinaki 2003]. Elastic support girdles that may give a proprioceptive input should be favored.

For such cases kyphoplasty is very promising, as it is currently the only minimally invasive treatment, apart from lordoplasty (see chapter 11), with which reduction of a fractured vertebral body can be achieved [Becker 2004], thus preventing the above-mentioned vicious circle from arising. Because of the very early and painless mobilization of the patient, efficient physiotherapy can be started much sooner and the patient can actively participate in the rehabilitation process at a very early stage. Corsets or braces are thus now unnecessary in the postoperative treatment.

Relation between kyphosis, the diaphragm and breathing

Schlaich [1998] measured the changes in vital capacity (VC) and forced expiratory volume (FEV1) in osteoporotic patients with a VBF, and found that the static changes of the spine led to distinct reduction of the both parameters. Respiration is our central "engine" and should not be forgotten in the treatment regimen. There are various possibilities for including respiration in the physiotherapeutic treatment. All patients can easily influence their breathing actively at home or in their spare time without having to spend a great deal of extra time. The nicest kind of "breathing therapy" is singing in a choir, which is, so to say, group pneumotherapy.

The diaphragm is not only our most important muscle for breathing but also a muscle that influences our posture (Fig. 106). As its insertions partly reach to L 3/4, it has a direct hold on the lumbar spine and hence on the complete spine. Most people have an elevated diaphragm and therefore have increased traction on the lumbar spine, even if they do not suffer from osteoporosis or other diseases. In addition, the diaphragm is interconnected with the iliopsoas muscle, hindering its ability to relax, and is therefore responsible for the hypertension of this muscle. The iliopsoas muscle is part of a chain of

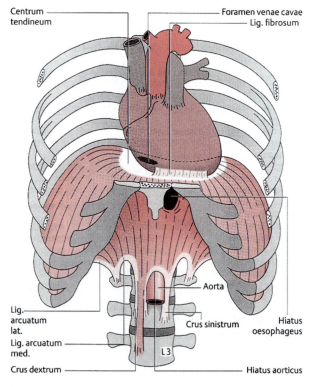

Fig. 106. Anatomical relationship of diaphragm – lumbar spine. From: *Strukturen und Funktionen begreifen* Vol. 1, Jutta Hochschild, Thieme, 2002, p. 84

flexors in our body; it keeps up a permanent flexion within the hip joints, i.e. a general inflected body posture. Thus the pattern "flexion" is activated and in consequence patients have great difficulty in actively straightening themselves up.

A therapy can only achieve long-term success if the whole system that is responsible for the deep muscular stabilization of the spine is active.

Relation between the abdominal wall and pelvic floor muscles, and the deep muscular stabilization system

The lungs, liver, heart, gastrointestinal system and other organs lie more or less freely within the thoracic and abdominal cavities. All these internal organs are strongly aqueous and have considerable weight. As is well known, liquid is not compressible. The "chamber" formed by the abdominal wall and pelvic floor muscles also represents a fluid-filled space. The walls of this abdominal chamber are cranially made up of the diaphragm, caudally of the muscles of the pelvic floor, and ventrally and laterally of the transversal abdominal muscle, which inserts dorsally in the thoracolumbar fascia (Fig. 107). For the first time in phylogenetic history, the pelvic floor and diaphragm have a supporting function; this is part of specific human development and cannot be found in this form in quadrupeds. The walls of the abdominal chamber, i.e. especially the pelvic floor muscles, diaphragm and abdominal transversal muscle, constitute a system that is responsible for the deep muscular stabilization of the spine, together with the monosegmental parts of the erector spinae muscles. If good functional capability of these muscles is provided, the abdominal chamber ensures the stability of the lumbar spine. This can be made clear by the phenomenon of weightlifters lifting loads several times their own body weight, after tightly girding the abdominal chamber for more stability.

In the case of malfunction (weakening or tension) of individual components responsible for deep muscular stabilization, the body tries to ensure stability through increased activation of the phylogenetically older muscles, especially of the flexors. Troubled with pain, patients adopt a stooped, bent position which often they cannot correct. This is intensified by the flexion of one group of muscles activating the contraction pattern "flexion" in the whole body, counteracting the ability to straighten up. The posture that develops is that of a dorsally tilted pelvis (neutralizing lumbar lordosis as a result), increased kyphosis of the cervicothoracic junction, shoulders pulled forward, the head pushed forward, and overstretched upper cervical joints. We also find this posture pattern in our osteoporotic patients.

How kyphosis and imbalance of the muscles are related

From the functional point of view the muscles have two main tasks: to ensure posture (statics) and to enable movement (dynamics) [Lewit 1998]. Although all muscles are involved in both tasks, the main role of the muscles of the trunk is to control upright posture. This function is primarily carried out by the tonic or fixation muscles, which produce less strength but can work for a long time without exhaustion. In contrast, the phasic muscles can develop great strength within a short time but cannot maintain it for long. If chronically overstressed (for example, if the deep stabilization system fails), the tonic muscles tend to develop increased tension

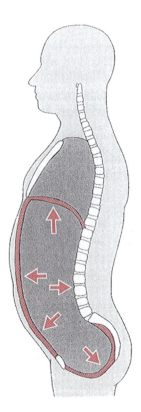

Fig. 107. Limiting structures of the abdominal chamber. From: *Topographie und Funktion des Bewegungssystems*, Michael Schünke, Thieme, 2000, p. 203

and in consequence shorten, whereas the phasic muscles tend to weaken. This results in a specific pattern of imbalance.

Among the group of muscles that tend to shorten are the short neck extensors, the descending part of the trapezius muscle, the major and minor pectoral muscles, the lumbar erector spinae, the iliopsoas muscle, the rectus femoris muscle, the ischiocrural muscles, the sural triceps muscle, the wrist flexors (e.g. the ulnar carpal flexor) and the finger flexors (e.g. the superficial digital flexor).

Among the group of muscles that tend to weaken are the deep neck extensors, the rectus abdominis muscle, the oblique abdominal muscle, the vastus medialis, lateralis, and intermedius muscles, the ascending part of the trapezius muscle, the rhomboid muscles and the thoracic erector spinae, the greatest and the middle gluteal muscle, the pelvic floor, the wrist extensors, the digital joints and the ankles.

The short autochthonous back muscles are decisive for an upright posture. They cannot be controlled by our free will or be activated consciously when there is a danger of falling; they work autonomously, e.g. as a reaction to a balance impulse, and can be trained only through sensomotoric exercise [Müller 2003].

Training and bone density

More than any other factor, physical stress affects the risk of fracture, and in manifold ways. In addition to reducing the frequency of falling [Robertson 2002], physical training has been shown in a large number of interventional studies to have positive effects on bone density in men and women of various ages [Bérard 1997]. Nevertheless, it has not definitely been proven that strength training has a positive effect on bone density and fracture risk, even though published results are encouraging [Sinaki 2002]. Despite an enormous number of studies, an ideal procedure that could maintain or increase bone density has still not been established.

It has been proven in animal experiments [Jarvinen 1998] that mechanical stress on the bone leads to reorganization of bone trabeculae without increasing bone density. Transferring this result to humans, it could mean that (strength-) training might lead to a lower fracture risk, although without improving bone density.

Scientific findings, however, clearly show that the objective often pursued – generating an increase of bone mass through strength training, thus reducing the fracture risk in older persons, especially those with osteoporosis – is not always appropriate [Papaioannou 2003]. Platen [2001] observes that, as a consequence of the reduced capacity and frequently bad general physical fitness in the affected age group, gaining bone mass is rather improbable because the stress stimuli, which must be set for a bone anabolic effect, cannot be achieved.

Instead, the appropriate age- and indication-specific aim for these patients must be sensomotoric training to improve coordination and balance. This reduces the danger of falling and lowers the fracture risk (Fig. 108).

Sensomotoric training

Sensomotoricity (a physiological term) or coordination (a sports-science term) is an ability based primarily on processes of intake and processing of information, and is dependent on

- a functioning perception,
- an intact nervous system,
- efficient skeletal muscles.

Laube [2000] observes that parts of the sensomotoric system can never be selectively (individually) addressed or put into function. Receptors cannot be trained on their own, only the whole functional (sensomotoric) system.

In practice this means that exercise programs that train the sensomotoric system as a whole need to be developed. This includes the task of reacting adequately to new, unexpected impulses, and doing so with a fast sequence of movements, thus optimizing the reflexive control of movement. Maintaining an upright posture during the sequence of movements is one of the main tasks of the deep muscular stabilization system (pelvic floor muscles, the diaphragm

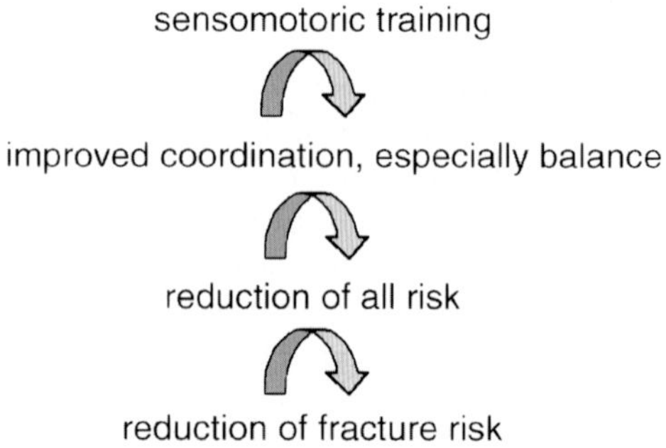

sensomotoric training

improved coordination, especially balance

reduction of all risk

reduction of fracture risk

Fig. 108. Age or indication specific objectives

and the transversal abdominal muscle constitute a system that is responsible for deep muscular stabilization of the spine, together with the monosegmental parts of the erector spinae muscles).

Sensomotoric training should therefore involve training the complete sensomotoric system, starting with the reception of information (perception), going on to performance of movement, and then storing the movement ("software development for the locomotor system"). This is the only possibility for exercising the short autochthonous back muscles as a part of the deep muscular stabilization system, as these can only be activated reflexively and work autonomously (e.g. reaction to a balance impulse). It allows unconsciously shifting the center of gravity of the body in order to stimulate postural responses of the deep muscular stabilization system.

Many (thousand) exercise repetitions are necessary to form new movement programs or to correct existing movement programs in the cerebellum [Meinel 1998]. This takes a long time and often involves the risk of stress reactions and even of harming. Furthermore, intervention studies with osteoporotic patients show that, especially in advanced age, the frequency of falling and the technique of falling correlate much more with an increased fracture rate than does bone density [Drinkwater 1995]. From this it can be inferred that, for reducing fracture incidents, improved sensomotoricity (balance) is more important than improved physical strength and the related increase of bone density.

This finding is also confirmed by Sinaki [2002] in a study with osteoporotic patients with distinctive kyphosis. The more insecure the patients are in their coordinative behavior, the more they profit from sensomotoric training regarding their equilibrium, which in turn has a positive effect on the risk of falling.

In analogy with studies on the prevention and treatment of backache, studies on osteoporosis almost without exception have dealt only with improvement of functional motor resources (strength, stamina, mobility) [Müller 2001]. Sensomotoric efficiency is, however, an essential predictor for the risk of falling, as it takes into account the interrelation between sensory control, cognitive representation, and motor control of posture (postural motoric system) and movement (directed motility), which is decisive for the occurrence of falling [Werle 1999]. The proprioceptive system is of great importance, as many older people with disorders of visual acuity and contrast sensitivity only lose their sense of bal-

ance if proprioception is also disturbed. According to Walter [2001], prevention of falling is one of the most important prophylactic issues concerning older people, in addition to incontinence, impairment of the sensory organs and threatening social isolation.

Sensomotoric training fulfils the following functions:

1. Creating a new movement program,
2. Automating movement.

Postoperative concepts with sensomotoric training

Sensomotoric training can be carried out with gymnastic apparatus that is very demanding for the equilibrium [Müller 2003]; for example, the aerostep®, the mini-trampoline and the gymnastics ball. Each apparatus can be used on its own but can also be sensibly combined with an exercise band or similar equipment. The sense of balance can also be trained during general activities of daily living.

aerostep®

The aerostep® is a gymnastic apparatus consisting of a flexible dual-chamber air cushion with either a smooth or a knobbled surface. During practice, the body must be permanently centered on the supporting area for gaining a "sense" of posture. The properties of the apparatus (unstable knobbled surface) enable effective training of the postural system, especially of its proprioceptive and tactile parts.

One characteristic of the aerostep® is that it is an ideal training device for home use. The aerostep® can be sensibly used even if only little space is available, unlike a gymnastics ball for example, and can be incorporated into everyday life, as simply standing on the device has a training effect. The device can be used when (Figs. 109–112):

– making a phone call,
– cleaning teeth,
– ironing,
– washing vegetables, peeling potatoes etc.,
– watching TV.

If patient and therapist use their imagination, they will surely come up with countless possibilities.

In a study of our own [Schwesig 2004], we showed that sensomotoric training on the aerostep® is able to improve the sensomotoric efficiency of

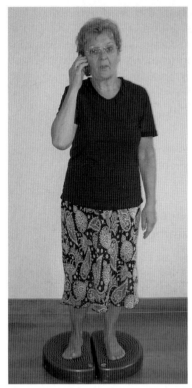
Fig. 109

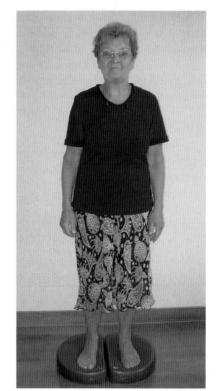
Fig. 110

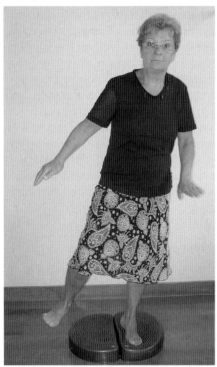
Fig. 111

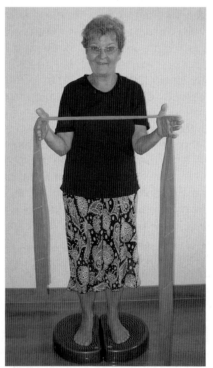
Fig. 112

Figs. 109–112. Exercises and activities that can be carried out on the aerostep®

older persons, especially those with osteoporosis. Significant improvements were found, particularly in static and dynamic ability to maintain equilibrium. These improvements were primarily based on adaptation within the peripheral vestibular system and on increased and more precise sagittal speed of movement. Furthermore, correlation with the variable "risk of falling" indicated a reduction of risk as a result of training on the aerostep®. The training program also had a positive influence on the state of health of the subjects, although it did not influence the quality of life. The training concept is not only objectively and subjectively effective; it is also highly practicable and has a high acceptance with users. Based on the results from these studies, it can be stated that there are almost no limits for the use of this training apparatus if set to use purposefully and skillfully.

Mini-trampoline

The advantage of the mini-trampoline over similar training forms on solid ground (e.g. skipping, running) lies in the fact that the braking distance on the trampoline is longer than on a hard surface. Thus peak loads and overstraining of the passive and the active support and movement system can be avoided. On the trampoline all body movements are primarily in the transverse plane while permanently and directly taking advantage of gravity [Schwesig 2004] (Fig. 113).

On the trampoline the body experiences two or three times the acceleration experienced in regular movements, but because the strain builds up relatively slowly the bodily structures are better able to cushion these greater forces, and as a result of the improved training effect the duration of treatment can be considerably shortened [Bayerlein 1997].

Furthermore, when exercising on the trampoline, the body must be centered within the support area when swinging/jumping on one spot. In doing so, the body experiences greater angular momentum around its horizontal axis than it does on solid ground. This causes corresponding shifting of the limbs and trunk. In addition, when jumping on the trampoline, neurophysiological straightening impulses are initiated. In particular, the vestibular activity (organ of equilibrium) and the monosynaptic stretch reflex in all the anti-gravity muscles are addressed. As a result of the permanent neurophysiological straightening impulses on the trampoline, the upright posture is stored in the motor memory and thus the basis for a new awareness of posture and movement is laid [Placht 1998].

Trampoline training primarily addresses the small monosegmental back extensors, which cannot be activated voluntarily and therefore can be trained only by reflex reaction. This is an important contribution to improvement of the functionality of the deep stabilization system and thus to better control of posture. The trampoline is therefore an ideal training device for patients with osteoporosis.

Furthermore, working with the trampoline also causes activation of other organ systems.

Depending on the intensity of training, the cardiovascular system is activated and in consequence the heart rate is increased. As with use of any other training equipment, it is also necessary to check the pulse and blood pressure regularly.

The activation of the cardiovascular system leads to an increased respiration rate and also to deeper breathing. This is the direct connection to the diaphragm (see above).

Positive effects on bone and muscle metabolism can be expected, as the result of changing gravitational forces during rebounding. Three bounces per second are normal and lead to a high-frequency activation of the receptors.

Our personal experience of several years with trampoline therapy has led us to see the mini-trampoline as an ideal training device, also for osteoporotic patients. Apart from positive factors such as the intensity and frequency of stimulus (up to 180 impulses/minute), there is a very positive influence on the motivation of patients. Even those who are critical and sceptical at the beginning of treatment "don't want to stop any more" after even a short while (Figs. 114, 115).

If trampoline therapy is used not only for sensomotoric training, it can simultaneously be used to stimulate bone anabolism. The qualities of the device mean that up to 3500 repetitions per training unit are no problem, which achieves positive effects

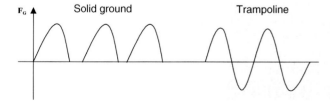

Fig. 113. Stress characteristics on solid ground and on the mini-trampoline

on bone metabolism. Kemmler [2003] states that the less the height of the stimulus, the higher the stimulus frequency should be. Thus, with the appropriate frequency, even a deformation of less than 1000 µΣ (microstrain) can have a positive influence on bone.

Note: The intensity of a stress stimulus (stimulus height, e.g. an axial compression) is typically measured as the relative deformation (strain) of the bone concerned and is given in microstrain (µΣ). 1000 µΣ is defined as change of length of 0.1%.

Outdoor training

Apart from integrating exercises into their everyday lives and into their personal surroundings, it is just as important that patients do not exercise only in artificial conditions, such as the gym, but also in natural surroundings. Crossing a street with high kerbs, getting on a bus or train and walking on uneven ground e.g. in a wood should be practised; however, only if patients know that they are able to get over these hurdles safely will they be prepared to face these situations. If patients lack the confidence to move outside their familiar environment they will quickly become socially isolated.

The pictures shown below of a playground visit are intended to illustrate one of the possibilities for outdoor activities (Figs. 116–119). Many patients with osteoporosis are grandparents and can use the time spent with their grandchildren positively for their health as well.

Is it realistic to expect a patient to exercise for 60 min 4–5 times a week? Do training programs with only one session per week make sense? There are no reliable data on what would be optimal train-

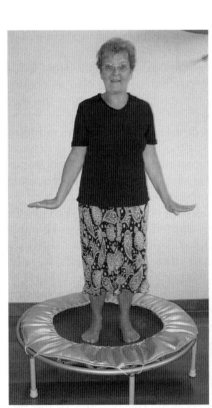
Fig. 114

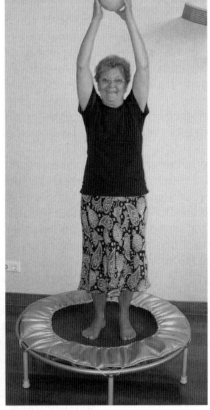
Fig. 115

Figs. 114, 115. Exercises that can be carried out on the mini-trampoline

ing, and in any case the frequency of training should meet both the following demands:

- Practicable and motivating for the patient
- Positive influence on bone parameters.

It is important that all patients taking part in a training program learn exercises that they can do on their own and carry out safely at home. The exercises should not require great additional effort such as changing clothes or assembling equipment, because only exercises that can be easily integrated into the daily routine will actually be done over a longer period.

All study results and considerations are of little use if the patient is not – or cannot be – motivated to take responsibility for exercising regularly. Doctors, therapists and family members are all asked to influence the patient positively in this respect. It is also important that the expectations set for the patient are realistic and practicable. Only very few patients will exercise daily for more than an hour, and keep up this practice over several years. The less the effort for the patient in terms of equipment, time and space to carry out the training program, the higher the probability that it will actually be done. Having fun is a big motivation factor, there-

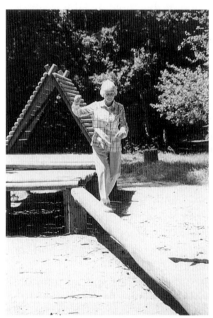

Fig. 116

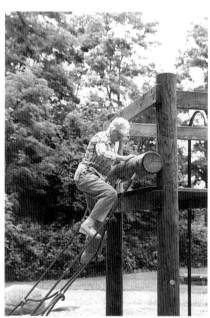

Fig. 117

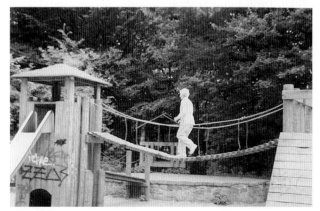

Fig. 118

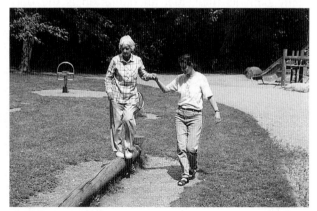

Fig. 119

Figs. 116–119. Outdoor activities

fore it is important to take the personal preferences of the patient into account. In this respect, a Viennese study [Kudlacek 1997] showed the positive effect that even a dance group for senior citizens had on the bone density of women with osteoporosis.

In the long term, patients will only regularly carry out training programs for which they are motivated.

Table 10. Muscle contraction pattern during in- and expiration

Muscular system	Inspiration	Expiration
Diaphragm	concentric	eccentric
Abdominal transverse muscle	eccentric	concentric
Pelvic floor	eccentric	concentric

Kyphosis and incontinence

We are deliberately addressing urinary incontinence (UI) in this context as its significance, especially for older people, our patients, should not be underestimated and has a strong influence on the quality of life.

The following data make this clear:

Epidemiology: Women are affected more often than men; there are considerably more data available concerning women than concerning men.

Among the total population, 12.6% suffer from urinary incontinence [Brähler 2004]: 6.1% of the 18–40 year olds, 9.5% of the 41–60 year olds, and already 30% of the over 60 year olds. At this age the number of affected men increases considerably and is comparable with the number of affected women. Unfortunately, only 15% of the persons affected get medical treatment.

Despite these clear figures, UI is often neglected by patients and physicians and is accepted as a normal part of aging. Often patients do not discuss the problem with their physician at all or only very late. It is important to address the problem of incontinence directly as, out of a sense of shame, patients often will not do this on their own. In addition, many patients think that an operation is the only possible treatment and thus keep quiet about the topic out of fear. Further, physicians who are not working in the field of gynecology or urology often know little about UI and therefore only hesitantly initiate diagnostic steps which are often insufficient.

Every occupational group dealing with older people should engage in this topic as UI has serious consequences:

Anxiety, depression, reduced social activity and shame often lead to isolation; UI is regarded as social death.

Incontinence is the second most frequent reason for nursing home admission and the principal cause for long-term care.

66% of incontinent women and 58% of incontinent men feel that their quality of life is lastingly restricted. Statistically, reduction of quality of life correlates significantly with the frequency and extent of incontinence, with impairment of sexuality and the necessity of carrying incontinence pads.

There are some risk factors for UI: age, BMI, births, hysterectomy [Madersbacher 2003] and, not least, kyphosis [Mattox 2000].

One form of incontinence has special relevance to patients suffering from kyphotic deformity of the spine.

Reflective incontinence is an insufficiency of the pelvic floor caused by a malfunctioning motor system [Rock 2003]. The main cause is a nonphysiological posture characterized by the following features: flexion of the spine – lowering of the thorax, extension of the pelvis – adduction of the hip – an-

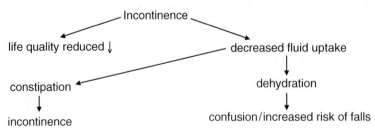

Fig. 120. Effects of incontinence

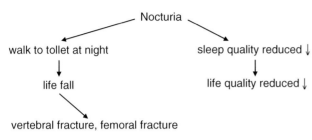

Fig. 121. Effects of nocturia

kle plantar flexion – lowered transverse arch of the foot.

Permanent inflection of the spine, whether lying, sitting or standing, reduces activity of the transverse abducting muscle, which in turn changes the activity of the pelvic floor muscles and in consequence their function within the bladder sphincter system [Sapsford 2001]. The intraabdominal pressure increases and thus also the pressure on the pelvic floor.

The transverse abdominal muscle connects the pelvis with the thorax and the spine, therefore the position of these parts of the trunk has an influence on the activity of the muscle and vice versa. It has been proven that the transverse abdominal muscle is considerably more active when the spine is stretched than when it is bent. The muscle and the pelvic floor act functionally together, as concentric activity of the transversal abducting muscle leads to activation of the pelvic floor and vice versa. An upright posture is therefore necessary for the physiological functioning of the pelvic floor, and its muscles are thus an integral part of the movement system and can be activated physiologically without isolated concentric activity having to be initiated. Nobody can or should have to think about trying to activate their pelvic floor 24 hours a day.

The cooperation of the transversal abducting muscle, the pelvic floor and the diaphragm can be explained logically by means of respiration physiology. During inhalation the diaphragm works concentrically and expands into the abdominal space. Here the pressure increases and the transversal abducting muscle and pelvic floor have to give way to the abdominal organs, i.e. both are working eccentrically. During exhalation it is the other way round. Malfunctioning of the diaphragm inevitably leads to impairment of the eccentric and concentric strength development of the pelvic floor (Table 10).

Patients sometimes try to overcome incontinence by restricting their fluid intake; this does not work and can lead to dehydration and a consequent state of confusion. This state can very easily lead to falling with the known far-reaching consequences.

Drinking very little also leads to constipation, where the increased demand for space within the true pelvis can induce overflow incontinence (Fig. 120).

Patients who suffer from nycturia risk falling every time they visit the toilet during the night. In addition, the quality of sleep is considerably reduced and eventually also the quality of life (Fig. 121).

Thus treating incontinence can also be seen as a prevention of falling.

In summary, incontinence can be treated and the earlier that therapy is started the better the chance of success; this can be up to 80%.

An upright posture, thus avoiding kyphotic malposition of the spine, is a pre-condition for adequate therapy or prophylaxis.

References

Bayerlein R (1997) Rebounding, Training und Therapie auf dem Minitrampolin – eine Einführung in das Rebounding und eine Anleitung für Patienten. Haug-Verlag

Becker S, Chavanne A, Meissner J, Bretschneider W, Ogon M (2004) Die minimal-invasive chirurgische Versorgung osteoporotischer Wirbelfrakturen mit Vertebroplastie und Kyphoplastie. J Miner Stoffwechs 11 [Suppl 1]: 4–7

Bérard A, Bravo G, Gauthier P (1997) Metaanalysis of the effectiveness of physical activity for the prevention of bone loss in postmenopausal women. Osteoporos Int 7: 331–7

Bös K, Brehm W (1998) Gesundheitssport – Ein Handbuch. Hofmann, Schorndorf

Brähler E (2004) Auch geringe Inkontinenz beeinflusst Lebensqualität. http://www.uni-protokolle.de/nachrichten/id/86798

Drinkwater BC, Mc Cloy H (1995) Research lecture: does physical activity play a role in preventing osteoporosis? Research Quarterly for Exercise and Sport 3: 197–206

Jarvinen TL, Kannus P, Sievanen H, et al (1998) Randomized controlled study of effects of sudden impact loading on rat femur. J Bone Miner Res 13: 1475–1482

Kemmler W, von Stengel S, Weineck J, Engelke K (2003) Empfehlungen für ein körperliches Training zur Verbesserung der Knochenfestigkeit: Schlussfolgerungen aus Tiermodellen und Untersuchungen an Leistungssportlern. Dtsch Z Sportmed 11: 306–16

Kudlacek S, Pietschmann P, Bernecker P, Resch H, Willvonseder R (1997) Effect of dancing on bone mass. Am J Phys Med Rehabil 76(6): 477–81

Laube, W (2001) Koordination und Sensomotorisches System in der Rehabilitation. In: Müller, Becker, Röhl, Seidel (Hrsg) Ausgewählte Aspekte der Physikalischen und Rehabilitativen Medizin. GFBB Verlag, Bad Kösen

Lewit K, Kolar P (1998) Funktionsstörung im Bewegungssystem – Verkettungen und Fehlprogrammierung. Krankengymnastik 8: 1346–52

Lynn SG, Sinaki M, Westerlind KC (1997) Balance characteristics of persons with osteoporosis. Arch Phys Med Rehabil 78: 273–77

Madersbacher S (2003) Prävalenz der weiblichen Harninkontinenz. J Urol Urogynäkol 1: 26–7

Mattox et al (2000) Abnormal spinal curvature and its relationship to pelvic organ prolapse. Am J Obstet Gynecol 183(6): 1381–4

Meinel K, Schabel G (1998) Bewegungslehre – Sportmotorik: Abriss einer Theorie der sportlichen Motorik unter pädagogischem Aspekt, 9. Aufl. Sportverlag, Berlin

Müller K, Schwesig R, Leuchte S, Riede D (2001) Koordinationstraining und Lebensqualität – Eine Längsschnittuntersuchung bei Pflegepersonal mit Rückenschmerzen. Gesundheitswesen 63: 609–18

Müller K, Schwesig R, Kreutzfeldt A, Becker S, Hottenrott K (2003) Das Rückenaktivprogramm. Meyer & Meyer, Aachen

Papaioannou A, Adachi JD, Winegard K, et al (2003) Efficacy of home-based exercise for improving quality of life among elderly women with symptomatic osteoporosis-related vertebral fractures. Osteoporos Int 14: 677–82

Placht W, Weiland A (1998) Die Proprioceptive Neuromuskuläre Trampolintherapie. Seminarinstitut W. Placht, Freiburg

Platen P (2001) Osteoporose – sind Prävention und Therapie durch Sport möglich? Bundesgesundheitsbl – Gesundheitsforsch – Gesundheitsschutz 44: 52–9

Robertson MC, Campbell AJ, Gardner MM, Devlin N (2002) Preventing injuries in older people by preventing falls: a meta analysis of individual-level data. J Am Geriatr Soc 50: 905–11

Rock C (2003) Beckenboden durch aufrechte Haltung. Physiopraxis 1: 2–5

Sapsford R (2001) Co-activation of the abdominal and pelvic floor muscles during voluntary exercises. Neurourol Urodyn 20: 31–42

Schlaich C, Minne HW, Bruckner T, et al (1998) Reduced pulmonary function in patients with osteoporotic fractures. Osteoporos Int 8: 261–7

Schwesig R, Müller K, Becker S, Kreutzfeldt A (2005) Entwicklung und Evaluation eines sensomotorischen Trainingsprogramms auf dem aerostep®. Bewegungstherapie und Gesundheitssport (In Druck)

Schwesig R, Scholz K, Kreutzfeldt A, Müller K, Becker S (2004) Sensomotorisches Training auf dem Minitrampolin. Bewegungstherapie und Gesundheitssport 20: 1–10

Sinaki M, Itoi E, Wahner HW, et al (2002) Stronger back muscles reduce the incidence of vertebral fractures: a prospective 10 year follow-up of postmenopausal women. Bone 30: 836–41

Sinaki M, Lynn SG (2002) Reducing the risk of falls through proprioceptive dynamic posture training in osteoporotic women with kyphotic posturing: a randomized pilot study. Am J Phys Med Rehabil 81(4): 241–6

Sinaki M (2003) Critical appraisal of physical rehabilitation measures after osteoporotic vertebral fracture. Osteoporos Int 14: 773–779

Skelton DA (2001) Effects of physical activity on postural stability. Age and Ageing 30 (S4): 33–9

Walter U, Schwarz FW (2001) Gutachten: Prävention im deutschen Gesundheitswesen, Medizinische Hochschule Hannover für die Kommission Humane Dienste (unveröffentlichtes Manuskript)

Werle J, Zimber A (1999) Sturzprophylaxe durch Bewegungssicherheit im Alter: Konzeption und Effektivitätsprüfung eines sensumotorischen Interventionsprogramms bei Osteoporose-Patientinnen. Z Gerontol Geriat 32: 348–57

Wolff I, Croonenborg van JJ, Kemper HCG, Kostense PJ, Twisk JWR (1999) The effect of exercise training programs on bone mass: a metaanalysis of published controlled trials in pre- and postmenopausal women. Osteoporos Int 9: 1–12

Appendix

The editors thank Mrs. B. Casteels (Vice President International, Health Policy & Government Relations, Kyphon International), for her help in summarising the current international reimbursement and coding status.

International coding of diseases according to ICD 10-GM 2004

Coding for osteoporosis

Main diagnosis ICD 10-GM 2004	Description
M80.08	Postmenopausal osteoporosis with pathological fracture
M80.18	Osteoporosis with pathological fracture after ovariectomy
M80.28	Inactivity osteoporosis with pathological fracture
M80.38	Osteoporosis with pathological fracture due to malabsorption after surgery
M80.48	Drug induced osteoporosis with pathological fracture
M80.58	Idiopathic osteoporosis with pathological fracture
M80.88	Other osteoporosis with pathological fracture

Coding for tumors

In the case of tumors the vertebral fracture has to be coded as a secondary diagnosis and the tumor as the main diagnosis.

Secondary diagnosis ICD 10-GM 2004	Description
M49.5-*	Vertebral body compression with elsewhere classified diseases
M49.5-4*	Thoracic region
M49.5-5*	Thoracolumbar region
M49.5-6*	Lumbar region
M49.5-7*	Lumbosacral region

Coding for trauma

In the case of several fractures, every single vertebra has to be coded.

Main diagnosis ICD 10-GM 2004	Description
S22.0-	Fracture of thoracic vertebra
S22.01	Th1 and Th2
S22.02	Th3 and Th4
S22.03	Th5und Th6
S22.04	Th7 and Th8
S22.05	Th9 and Th10
S22.06	Th11 and Th12
S32.0-	Fracture of lumbar vertebra
S32.01	L1
S32.02	L2
S32.03	L3
S32.04	L4
S32.05	L5

Reimbursement codes per country (in alphabetical order)

Austria

MEL	Description
1255	CT-assisted reduction and filling of vertebral body with balloon catheter (kyphoplasty). Coding = 1 session

This MEL is subject to the following conditions: "For the clearance of MEL 1255 the units must be approved by the regional health commission. Prerequisite for the approval is a center for spine surgery at the hospital.

The MEL code tracks to MEL group 01.17: Minimal Invasive intervention in the Spine. The relative weights for this MEL group 4.068 points for the intervention + 1.017 points for the hospitalisation =

total of 5.085 points or ± 5.100 Euros. This is the flexible part paid to the hospital on top of the fixed funding by the Länder as global hospital budget.

Belgium

No reimbursement exists for Balloon Kyphoplasty yet.

Some private insurances reimburse the traumatic cases (work accidents);

The Belgian expert centre (KCE) assessed Balloon Kyphoplasty and issued a positive guidance in November 2006.

France

Public hospitals (AP)

Balloon Kyphoplasty can be financed by capped hospital budget (référencement) and according to the GHS (French DRGs):

- Spine intervention without complication: 3 902.96 €
- Spine intervention with complication: 6 187.79 €

Balloon Kyphoplasty can be financed by local innovation budgets

Balloon Kyphoplasty can be funded under the STIC budget as from 2007. The DOH has allocated a specific budget for 4 studies on Balloon Kyphoplasties for 2 years:

- Randomized study on fresh osteoporotic vertebral fractures: BKP versus vertebroplasty versus conventional medical management with a brace (100 patients in each group).
- Randomized study on old osteoporotic vertebral fractures: BKP versus vertebroplasty (100 patients in each groups).
- Randomized study on traumatic fractures A1 and A2: BKP versus vertebroplasty (100 patients in each group) with the KyphX cement.
- Observational study on traumatic vertebral fracture (A3, B1 and C1) BKP + posterior open surgery: 50 BKP with the KyphX cement.

Private hospitals

Balloon Kyphoplasty can be financed within the framework of a local innovation budget.

File for national reimbursement was submitted beginning 2007 for the following indications:

- Intensive and persistent pain treatment and vertebral deformation correction linked with osteoporoses vertebral fractures with the KyphX cement.
- Intensive and persistent pain treatment linked with osteolytic vertebral fractures with the KyphX cement.
- Reduction and stabilization of A3 burst vertebral fractures: BKP + posterior open surgery with the KyphOs.

The private insurances reimburse to the patients the part of hospital expenses not funded by the Public Health Insurances.

Germany

In Germany, all inpatient acute-care hospital services are financed according to the G-DRG system. The fees of the G-DRG system apply equally to both private and social health insurers.

The 2006 version of the G-DRG system contains 878 codes (the 2007 version contains 954 codes) that group hospital episodes according to the primary diagnosis upon admission to a hospital and the procedures used during treatment. Each DRG is associated with a "relative weight" that is supposed to reflect the amount of resource utilization associated with a DRG in relation to the average resource utilization of all hospital cases (for which the relative weight is set at unity).

To calculate the amount of payment associated with a DRG, its relative weight is multiplied by the "base rate" of a hospital. The base rate is supposed to reflect the average cost of a hospital case in monetary terms. Currently, the DRG system is moving from individual base rates for each hospital to payment based on state-wide base rates.

Although earlier versions of the G-DRG system contained different DRGs for kyphoplasty that depended on the primary diagnosis, in the 2006 and 2007 versions, one DRG code covers all patients who are admitted to the hospital for treatment of the fracture of a vertebral body and are treated using kyphoplasty, regardless of the underlying reason for the fracture. As long as the procedural code OPS 5-839.a_ ("implant of material in vertebrae following height restoration´") is the main procedure, inpatient care for a vertebral fracture will be paid for by private and social health insurers according to the DRG code I09, "fusion of a vertebra".

Appendix

DRGs G01Z I79Z 2005	Description
5-839.a-	Implantation of material into a vertebral body with preceding reduction, incl. kyphoplasty
5-839.a-0	1 segment
5-839.a-1	2 segments
5-839.a-2	3 segments
5-839.a-3	More than 3 segments
Additional code 5-986	Application of minimal invasive techniques

This code is broken down into three sub-codes, I09A, I09B and I09C, with A representing treatment with the most resource utilization (e.g. due to two or more co-morbidities) and C treatment with the least amount of resource utilization.

Assuming a base rate of € 2,900, the level of payment associated with the 2006 DRGs for kyphoplasty are given below:

2006

I09A: relative weight 4.168 $\Rightarrow$ € 12,087.20
I09B: relative weight 3.209 $\Rightarrow$ € 9,306.10
I09C: relative weight 2.306 $\Rightarrow$ € 6,687.40

The relative weights for 2007 have increased slightly over their values in 2006 for the group I09A (by 4%) and only minimally for the DRGs I09B and I09C (by 1.3% and 0.22% respectively). The levels of payment in 2007 for each DRG are given below assuming a base rate of € 2,900.

2007

I09A: relative weight 4.333 $\Rightarrow$ € 12,565.70
I09B: relative weight 3.251 $\Rightarrow$ € 9,427.90
I09C: relative weight 2.311 $\Rightarrow$ € 6,701.90

2008

I09A: relative weight 4.727 $\Rightarrow$ € 13,708.30
I09B: relative weight 3.240 $\Rightarrow$ € 9,396.00
I09C: relative weight 2.694 $\Rightarrow$ € 7,812.60
I09D: relative weight 2.237 $\Rightarrow$ € 6,487.30

Greece

The balloon kyphoplasty procedure and devices are reimbursed in Greece.

Italy

In Italy, the procedures are financed by DRGs.

Balloon Kyphoplasty can be financed by different DRGs depending on the diagnosis and complications of the patient.

The procedure ICD-9-CM-2002 code used for BKP is:
- Code 78.49: other restoring treatments/plasty on bone/vertebra.
- The BKP procedure is generally provide as inpatient treatment (length of stay 2 days).
- DRG 233: other treatment on musculoskeletal system with complication (average of € 6,980).
- DRG 234: other treatment on musculoskeletal system without complication (average of € 3,300).
- The DRG's tariffs could change in a range of ± 10% depending regions and Hospital.
- No extra reimbursement is provided for multi-level treatment.

Netherlands

Balloon Kyphoplasty can be financed within the free part of the hospital budget under code 05.11.1395.223. The amount for this DBC is for one level. For each extra level, an additional 50% of this payment can be added.

The hospital also has the possibility to ask for a specific budget for this innovative treatment. This is already the case in several hospitals in the Netherlands. A request for a specific DBC for balloon kyphoplasty has been introduced.

Ontario

Balloon Kyphoplasty is funded in Ontario. Payment for the procedure (medical act) is under the following codes:

- #N583 Kyphoplasty (balloon tamp and injection of bone cement)
- as sole procedure, first level 969.00
- #E392-kyphoplasty combined with any other procedure
- first level, to other procedure. . . . . .add 510.00
- #E393-kyphoplasty, each additional level, to N583 or
- E392 . . . . .add 510.00
- #E381-intra-operative, diagnostic or physiological neuro
- monitoring, to N583 or E392 . . . . . .add 179.30

These codes give the surgeons a total of Ca$ 1,148.30 for the first level of BKP and $ 510 for each additional level (payment for the surgical procedure).

Biopsy with Needle is coded under Z940 at $ 142.80. This code can be billed additionally to the balloon kyphoplasty code when a biopsy is performed during the Balloon kyphoplasty procedure.

The devices are reimbursed separately.

South Africa

The South African private insurers reimburse Balloon kyphoplasty.

Spain

In Spain, balloon Kyphoplasty is financed out of the global budget of the hospital or by private Insurers.

Switzerland

The Swiss Home Office (Eidgenössisches Department des Inneren) has temporarily added kyphoplasty to the health insurance scheme as of January 1st, 2005, valid until December 31st, 2007. The following benefits are included:

Acute painful vertebral body fractures that don't respond to treatment with analgesics, and which show a deformity that needs to be corrected; the following indications according to the guidelines of the Swiss Society for Spinal Surgery of September 23, 2004 must be given for the applicability of the insurance scheme for kyphoplastic treatment:

- 15° thoracic kyphosis or 10° lumbar kyphyosis or
- At least 1/3 height reduction of the vertebra in comparison with adjacent vertebrae;
- Fracture not older than 8 weeks or persisting painful fracture (VAS persisting > 5) older than 8 weeks;
- Pain must be caused by the fracture;
- Vertebral compression fracture caused by tumor.

Furthermore the operation must be documented over a two year period with follow-up examinations.

A Swiss balloon kyphoplasty register with examination sheets (MEMdoc of April 28, 2005) is available.

The operation can only be carried out by a surgeon certified either by the Swiss Society for Spinal Surgery, the Swiss Society for Orthopaedics, or the Swiss Society for Neurosurgery. These three societies have, amongst others, initiated an evaluation programme for this service; the results will serve as a basis for the decisions to be taken in 2007. Initially this service is limited to three years.

Until now there isn't a specific reimbursement number in the Swiss reimbursement catalogue (Spitalleistungskatalog) or in the Health Care Benefit Regulation (Krankenpflegeleistungsverordnung).

The level of funding is in principle free and will depend on the agreements the hospital made (can be DRG-like or fee for service).

BKP is funded in Switzerland for traumatic patients by the accident insurances.

Turkey

The balloon kyphoplasty procedure and devices are reimbursed in Turkey.

UK

Public Sector (NHS)

The Department of Health (DoH) has issued Balloon Kyphoplasty with it's own specific code:

V445: Balloon Kyphoplasty for fracture of spine. This code will continue to map to HRG R03 for the 2007/08 fiscal year (see Table 11).

Private Sector

The BCWA (committee for private medical insurance providers UK) has issued Balloon Kyphoplasty with its own specific code:

Table 11

HRG code	HRG name	Elective spell tariff (£)	Elective long stay trimpoint (days)	Non-elective spell tariff (£)	Non-elective long stay trimpoint (days)	Per day long stay payment (for days exceeding trimpoint) (£)
R03	Decompression and effusion for degenerative spinal disorders	5,100	13	6,984	48	248

Appendix

XR542: Balloon Kyphoplasty for fracture of spine. This code went live on the 1st of November 2006 and will be reimbursed by the major private medical insurance providers.

Under this code the surgeon will be paid an average of £ 1,400 for one level.

USA

Medicare and Medicaid Services (CMS) issued a recommendation as part of the 2005 Inpatient Prospective Payment System (IPPS) Rule that allows a unique ICD-9 code for balloon kyphoplasty, which is 81.66. This code permits payment under five potential DRG codes. Balloon kyphoplasty procedure (not including the medical act) is covered under the following DRGs:

DRG 233: Musculosceletal System and Connective Tissue or Procedures with complications or co-morbidities.
DRG 234: Musculosceletal System and Connective Tissue or Procedures without complications or co-morbidities.
DRG 442: Other OR Procedures for Injuries, with cc.
DRG 443: Other OR Procedures for Injuries, without cc.
DRG 486: Other OR Procedures for multiple significant trauma.

Since January 1, 2006, the following CPT codes are effective for physician reimbursement for kyphoplasty (see Table 12).

Using the newly published fee schedule, the adjusted Medicare payment to physicians for their professional services is expected to range from approximately $ 565 to $ 778 for a single-level balloon kyphoplasty procedure with fluoroscopy and approximately $ 872-1,175 for a two-level balloon kyphoplasty procedure with fluoroscopy. These ranges reflect that Medicare payment rates are adjusted to account for geographic variations in practice expenses and malpractice insurance costs.

The authors cannot guarantee or promise coverage or payment for any products or any procedures. Such determinations are made based on, including but not limited to, individual patient conditions, the Health Insurance schemes in place and the patient's insurances.

This reimbursement update represents at the time of writing the author's best knowledge/efforts to include accurate, reliable and up to date information. The authors do not make any warranties or representations, express or implied, as to the accuracy, reliability, correctness and completeness of the content of the reimbursement update and assumes in this respect no liability or responsibility for any inaccuracies, errors, omissions, misstatement and incompleteness nor can the authors be held liable for any miscoding of the balloon kyphoplasty procedures.

Table 12

CPT Code	Description	2006 RVUs	Unadjusted payment
22523	Percutaneous vertebral augmentation, including cavity creation (fracture reduction including biopsy when performed) using mechanical device, one vertebral body, unilateral or bilateral cannulation (e.g. kyphoplasty); thoracic	16.29	$ 589.32
22524	Percutaneous vertebral augmentation, including cavity creation (fracture reduction including biopsy when performed) using mechanical device, one vertebral body, unilateral or bilateral cannulation (e.g. kyphoplasty); lumbar	15.61	$ 564.72
22525	Each additional thoracic or lumbar vertebral body (List separately in addition to code for primary procedure)	7.47	$ 270.24
76012	Radiologic supervision and interpretation, percutaneous vertebroplasty or vertebral augmentation including cavity creation, per vertebral body; under fluoroscopic guidance	1.88	$ 68.01
76013	Radiologic supervision and interpretation, percutaneous vertebroplasty or vertebral augmentation including cavity creation, per vertebral body; under CT guidance	1.93	$ 69.82

SpringerMedicine

Walter Hruby (ed.)

Digital (R)Evolution in Radiology

Bridging the Future of Health Care

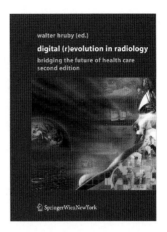

2., revised and enlarged edition.
2006. XVI, 379 pages. Numerous figures, partly in colour.
Hardcover **EUR 160,–**
ISBN 978-3-211-20815-1

According to a statement of Gordon Moore computer performance doubles every 18 months. So it is not surprising that the "half-time" of modern computers is rapidly decreasing. Increasing demands of public health for radiology together with a rapid development of information technology and innovations result in a digital environment, where thorough guidance is necessary. This book is such a solid guidance for radiologists and other medical staff working in this field.

The second edition has been brought up-to-date, revised and new aspects have been incorporated that focus on the synergy that results from the integration of digital systems used in radiology such as image fusion, "functional" imaging, electronic patient records and health networks, etc. It is intended for radiologists and all other physicians, as well as technicians, scientists, IT-experts, health care providers and health maintenance organisations. The IT-market now has changed so much that Integrated Health Care Enterprise becomes reality.

SpringerWienNewYork

P.O. Box 89, Sachsenplatz 4–6, 1201 Vienna, Austria, Fax +43.1.330 24 26, books@springer.at, springer.at
Haberstraße 7, 69126 Heidelberg, Germany, Fax +49.6221.345-4229, SDC-bookorder@springer-sbm.com, springer.com
P.O. Box 2485, Secaucus, NJ 07096-2485, USA, Fax +1.201.348-4505, service@springer-ny.com, springer.com
All errors and omissions excepted. Recommended retail price. Net-price subject to local VAT.

SpringerMedicine

J. Manninger et al. (Eds.)
Internal fixation of femoral neck fractures
An Atlas

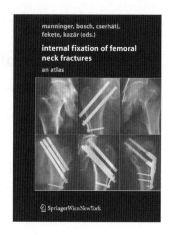

2007. XIX, 310 p. 242 illus.
Hardcover. **EUR 134,95**
ISBN 978-3-211-68583-9

Femoral neck fractures occur primarily in the elderly population, and nowadays arthroplasty is chosen most frequently as a treatment solution. In the era of financial restrictions in health care system non-invasive internal fixation is an attractive choice, because in addition to the lower immediate costs the rehabilitation period might also be shorter. In this illustrated atlas the authors deal with epidemiological aspects, anatomical and biomechanical specialities of the given region, diagnostic and management potentials, satisfactory both for orthopaedic and trauma specialists.

By means of presenting minimally invasive technique step-by-step, and their own results, the aim is to persuade the reader that the ratio of complications remarkably can be diminished by urgent surgery, based on selective indication criteria. Aspects of postoperative treatment and rehabilitation are also clarified in details. The research team under the guidance of Professor Manninger collected experiences of 50 years.

SpringerWienNewYork

P.O. Box 89, Sachsenplatz 4–6, 1201 Vienna, Austria, Fax +43.1.330 24 26, books@springer.at, springer.at
Haberstraße 7, 69126 Heidelberg, Germany, Fax +49.6221.345-4229, SDC-bookorder@springer-sbm.com, springer.com
P.O. Box 2485, Secaucus, NJ 07096-2485, USA, Fax +1.201.348-4505, service@springer-ny.com, springer.com
All errors and omissions excepted. Recommended retail price. Net-price subject to local VAT.

SpringerMedicine

Bernhard Schaller (Ed.)

Imaging of Carotid Artery Stenosis

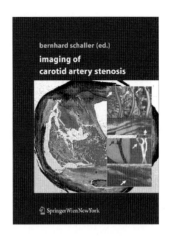

2007. VI, 273 p. 86 illus., 50 in color.
Hardcover. **EUR 198,–**
ISBN 978-3-211-32332-8

Stroke is the third leading cause of death and carotid atherosclerosis is the leading cause of embolic stroke. In recent years, the need for a more detailed analysis of atherosclerotic plaques has been stressed. Information beyond the degree of narrowing of the vessel lumen seems to be desirable and there is considerable demand for diagnostic procedures that specifically identify rupture-prone, vulnerable plaques as the most frequent cause of sudden ischemic events. This atlas is an up-to-date reference work on imaging in carotid artery stenosis written by internationally renewed experts.

The authors take the reader step by step through illustrated descriptions of state-of-the-art imaging techniques that they have helped to develop, and demonstrate that these techniques are crucial in the management of patients. This book covers all facets of imaging in carotid artery stenosis and gives an outlook to future aspects. The 'take-home-messages' at the end of each chapter are a quick help in daily practice.

SpringerWienNewYork

P.O. Box 89, Sachsenplatz 4–6, 1201 Vienna, Austria, Fax +43.1.330 24 26, books@springer.at, springer.at
Haberstraße 7, 69126 Heidelberg, Germany, Fax +49.6221.345-4229, SDC-bookorder@springer-sbm.com, springer.com
P.O. Box 2485, Secaucus, NJ 07096-2485, USA, Fax +1.201.348-4505, service@springer-ny.com, springer.com
All errors and omissions excepted. Recommended retail price. Net-price subject to local VAT.

Springer and the Environment

WE AT SPRINGER FIRMLY BELIEVE THAT AN INTER-national science publisher has a special obligation to the environment, and our corporate policies consistently reflect this conviction.

WE ALSO EXPECT OUR BUSINESS PARTNERS – PRINTERS, paper mills, packaging manufacturers, etc. – to commit themselves to using environmentally friendly materials and production processes.

THE PAPER IN THIS BOOK IS MADE FROM NO-CHLORINE pulp and is acid free, in conformance with international standards for paper permanency.